A Writer's Toolkit for Occupational Therapy and Health Care Professionals

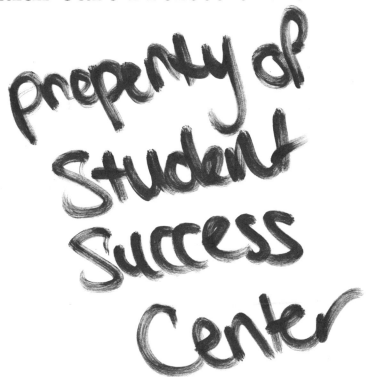

A Writer's Toolkit
for Occupational Therapy
and Health Care Professionals

An Insider's Guide to Writing, Communicating, and Getting Published

Edited by
Rondalyn V. Whitney, PhD, OT/L,
and Christina A. Davis

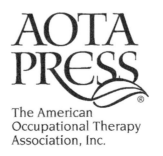

The American
Occupational Therapy
Association, Inc.

AOTA Centennial Vision
We envision that occupational therapy is a powerful, widely recognized, science-driven, and evidence-based profession with a globally connected and diverse workforce meeting society's occupational needs.

AOTA Mission Statement
The American Occupational Therapy Association advances the quality, availability, use, and support of occupational therapy through standard-setting, advocacy, education, and research on behalf of its members and the public.

AOTA Staff
Frederick P. Somers, *Executive Director*
Christopher M. Bluhm, *Chief Operating Officer*

Christina A. Davis, *Director, AOTA Press*
Ashley Hofmann, *Development/Production Editor*
Victoria Davis, *Digital/Production Editor*

Beth Ledford, *Director, Marketing*
Jennifer Folden, *Marketing Specialist*
Amanda Fogle, *Marketing Specialist*

American Occupational Therapy Association, Inc.
4720 Montgomery Lane
Bethesda, MD 20814
Phone: 301-652-AOTA (2682)
TDD: 800-377-8555
Fax: 301-652-7711
www.aota.org
To order: 1-877-404-AOTA or store.aota.org

Disclaimers
This publication is designed to provide accurate and authoritative information in regard to the subject matter covered. It is sold or distributed with the understanding that the publisher is not engaged in rendering legal, accounting, or other professional service. If legal advice or other expert assistance is required, the services of a competent professional person should be sought.
—*From the Declaration of Principles jointly adopted by the American Bar Association and a Committee of Publishers and Associations*

It is the objective of the American Occupational Therapy Association to be a forum for free expression and interchange of ideas. The opinions expressed by the contributors to this work are their own and not necessarily those of the American Occupational Therapy Association.

ISBN 978-1-56900-311-4

Library of Congress Control Number: 2013937734

Cover design by Jennifer Folden, AOTA Press, Bethesda, MD
Text design by Naylor Design, Washington, DC
Composition by Maryland Composition, Laurel, MD
Printed by Automated Graphic Systems, White Plains, MD

Contents

Boxes, Figures, and Tables

BOXES

FIGURES

TABLES

Preface

Do one thing every day that scares you.

—ELEANOR ROOSEVELT (N.D.)

During our combined 40 years of working with health care writing, we have encountered many intelligent people who have had technical difficulty with communicating and who have lacked the confidence to share their knowledge and experiences with an audience. Part of this can be explained by the decreasing emphasis on writing and communicating that has crept into the U.S. education system over the past generation and part by the high-level and often inaccessible writing that appears from experts in a field, who tend to shroud their core message in jargon and run-on sentences. This book's editors—a well-published occupational therapy clinician, researcher, and educator and an experienced health care publisher—know that it doesn't have to be this way. We have long imagined a book that would present writing as both an important and attainable skill for occupational therapy students during education and fieldwork and for occupational therapy professionals throughout a career.

Professional writing and communicating are more craft than art, starting with a creative and thoughtful concept that requires the author to give that concept substance. Even art has a structure. Artists use organization to define their inspiration, choose the right tools and techniques, schedule time to work on their project, and refine their processes and skills to complete a finished product. A blacksmith selects and hones a piece of metal, forging it into a sword or sculpture. A flutist learns, through practice, how to create the perfect haunting note by controlling the just-right tension while exhaling precisely. Similarly, writers learn to control superfluous thought and build a tool chest of words and skills to precisely communicate their intent.

This book will help writers and communicators step over the threshold from novice to writer to teacher and along the journey develop confidence, tools, and skills. Chapters are organized by graduating steps to help readers acquire more complex skills as they move through the sections. This book is designed to teach, inform, inspire, and empower readers to fulfill their writing and communicating ambitions, whether academic, professional, personal, or scholarly. Readers can start anywhere, addressing their own problem areas and concerns.

How to Use This Book

While it is true that reading a book on writing won't make you a great writer, it can offer some ideas about how to solve the problems that have blocked your path and thwarted your aspirations. Writing and communicating require organization, habits, routines, and rituals that expand your ability to express and share your ideas with others. Most of all, they require confidence in your abilities.

In **"Part I: Gaining Confidence,"** the authors introduce the internal dialogue of a writer and help you find your own voice. In Chapter 1, Donna Costa welcomes you to the world of writing by encouraging you to reflect on the potential barriers to writing with confidence. In Chapter 2, Elizabeth Cara shows how writing as an occupation can be considered through the lens of aggregate activities, habits, routines, and even rituals. In Chapter 3, Suzanne M. Peloquin gently takes readers by the hand in search of their own "authentic voice."

In **"Part II: Getting Started,"** chapters review the foundational components of writing. In Chapter 4, Rondalyn V. Whitney reviews basic organizational strategies to revision techniques to tone and style. Robert G. Hess, Jr., and Lisa Foulke give a publisher's view of how to successfully navigate the submission process in Chapter 5. In Chapter 6, Sharon A. Gutman provides salient instruction for how to collaborate on team projects. Christina A. Davis completes this section in Chapter 7 with an explanation of an often-overlooked ingredient of success—following a publisher's preferred writing style.

In **"Part III: Writing for Your Audience,"** chapters cover various types of publications and their audiences. In Chapter 8, Alison B. Miller offers critical advice for overcoming the mental self-talk standing between you and your thesis or dissertation. In Chapter 9, Catherine Foster and Luther G. Kalb explain how to present research findings with elegance. Whether writing a systematic review or a grant proposal or writing about a unique practice in your setting or documenting treatment, Marian Arbesman, Leonard G. Trujillo, Winifred Schultz-Krohn, and Jerilyn (Gigi) Smith provide field-tested guidance for readers in Chapters 10, 11, 12, and 13, respectively. In Chapter 14, Davis offers advice for those who want to write professionally.

You likely are or will be one of the many professionals who are expanding their communications repertoire to include presentations, virtual meetings, and social media. **"Part IV: Writing and Communicating in the New Media"** provides advice for speaking to a crowd. Whitney shares tips for creating and delivering a presentation (Chapter 15), and Brent Braveman offers learned wisdom about conducting online meetings with multiple stakeholders (Chapter 16). Fran Babiss defines the ground rules for proper social conduct in a virtual community (Chapter 17).

"Part V: Sharing Your Writing Knowledge" is important, because not everyone who teaches writing is a writer, nor are writers necessarily natural teachers. In Chapter 18, Whitney offers advice for teaching gathered from years behind the lectern, and in Chapter 19, Karen Jacobs and Nancy MacRae remind readers to "pay it forward" by mentoring others.

Conclusion

As we feel masterful in the pursuit of an occupation, it grows to be deeply satisfying. Mary Reilly (1962) said it best: "Man, through the use of his hands, as they are energized by mind and will, can influence the state of his own health" (p. 1). Writing, when energized by the mind, controlled by the will, and tempered by practice and diligence, can promote health as the writers' insights and discoveries are shared through their published texts. In addition, people can be healed by the act of reading powerful words. And good writing and communicating can lead to better grades on or more timely completion of assignments. We hope that this work will help you meet your goals, whether academic, professional, personal, or scholarly.

REFERENCES

Reilly, M. (1962). Occupational therapy can be one of the great ideas of 20th-century medicine (1961 Eleanor Clarke Slagle Lecture). *American Journal of Occupational Therapy, 16*, 1–9.

Roosevelt, E. (n.d.) *Eleanor Roosevelt quotes.* Available online at http://www.goodreads.com/author/quotes/44566.Eleanor_Roosevelt

Acknowledgments

The writers who contributed to this book each enthusiastically stepped forward when asked to share their knowledge with future aspiring writers and their peers. This book is a gift from the authors to you, the readers—a gift that they hope you will use to write and communicate well. We thank them for their selfless generosity.

We would be remiss if we did not acknowledge some of the other individuals who made this book happen.

Personally, my contribution to this effort would not have been feasible without my coeditor Christina Davis' vision and quiet, tenacious commitment to excellence; our production editor Steve Pazdan's undauntable spirit; or the encouragement and honest feedback of the students in the advanced writing seminars I had the pleasure to teach while in the College of Applied Sciences and Arts at San José State University. I learned from my students that whereas writing is powerful, awaking the writer in others is humbling and very often transformative for both teacher and student. My colleagues in the Department of Occupational Therapy at University of the Sciences provided encouragement for this work. In addition, I wish to thank Wendy Fox, MOT, OTR/L; Claudia Hilton, PhD, MBA, OTR/L, FAOTA; and Paula Kramer, PhD, OTR/L, FAOTA, for reviewing earlier drafts of this book.

I want to acknowledge two of my own occupational therapy writing "heroes": Dr. Suzanne M. Peloquin and Dr. Elizabeth Cara. Peloquin's work has always inspired and moved the profession forward, as she artistically interweaves scientific writing and heartfelt prose, steadfastly reaching for hands and hearts as her life's work, cohesively illustrated in her scholarship. Cara exemplifies how engaging in the habits and routines of a writer produces written testimony to the courage of others. Finally, I acknowledge my family. My husband, Bill, is my rock and my life's greatest blessing. He has picked up my share of our family's chores for more than 21 years when I have pushed against writing deadlines, yet he does so with great heart and loving encouragement. My two sons, Zac and Alex, have stretched my heart, requiring me to expand my own sensory vocabulary in the futile attempt to express the overflowing joy I have from being their mom and watching them live their lives with such fantastic exuberance.

—R.V.W.

Without the amazing patience and forbearance of Rondalyn Whitney and the other authors, this book would not have happened. K. Hyde Loomis skillfully edited this work, and Steve Pazdan kept it going when I could not. My inspiration was provided by Kate Kelly, Linda Beebe, and Nancy Winchester, who have impressed on me for the past quarter-century that scholarly, technical, and medical publishing, while not as glamorous or lucrative as, say, the latest teenage vampire saga, is the most important publishing, as it can actually save lives. Therefore, doing it right is paramount. Part of doing it right is making sure significant research results are clearly shared and novel solutions find the widest audience. It is my hope that occupational therapy professionals and students, who are some of the most thoughtful and entrepreneurial people I have ever met, will find the confidence to tell their stories and the clarity to make them heard.

—C.A.D.

Gaining
Confidence

PART I

So You Want to Write? Facing the Challenge With Confidence

DONNA COSTA, DHS, OTR/L, FAOTA

And by the way, everything in life is writable about if you have the outgoing guts to do it, and the imagination to improvise. The worst enemy to creativity is self-doubt.

— Sylvia Plath (1982, p. 83)

I t's 3:00 a.m., and you're staring at a blank computer screen with a deadline looming in a few hours. How do you get past that screen?

You have an idea that you think is a good one, and you'd like to tell someone. How will you turn your idea into a written masterpiece, or even an adequate paper?

You are asked to coauthor an article, or copresent at a conference, or coteach a workshop. How do you get the confidence to respond "Yes, I can do that!" when asked to collaborate?

You are thinking about accepting your first teaching position but have heard that the "publish or perish" pressure is terrible. You love to teach and want to give back to a profession that has meant so much to you, but how will you face the challenges in this incredible opportunity?

You are afraid that your creativity has dried up and that you'll never write again, despite having written two books, four book chapters, and dozens of articles. How do you rediscover your inner writer?

The above scenarios are familiar to everyone who writes, whether they are students, therapists, professors, researchers, or seasoned authors. The challenge of taking pen to paper or fingers to keyboard is precisely that—a challenge. Professor Wendy Belcher (2009) wrote about "writing dysfunction" and her experiences teaching a writing course at the University of California, Los Angeles, for 10 years. She described her own college experience of repeatedly submitting papers to professors and not understanding what they wanted from her. At the time, she thought that only she faced this dilemma and that other students knew how to write the papers their instructors were assigning. She believed that other students possessed confidence that she did not have:

> I began to suspect that everyone but me knew how to organize their time, do their research, and write successful papers. I managed to muddle through, but I felt like an imposter—I believed a real scholar would know exactly what to do. It never occurred to me to wonder how she would know or where she would have found out what to do. (p. 186)

Only years after earning her doctorate did she come to realize that her peers all faced the same issues.

Where does one learn confidence in writing? Unfortunately, this confidence is not usually gained during one's college education. Students—undergraduates, graduates, postdocs—are expected to write but are given little, if any, instruction on writing. Professors' feedback on assigned papers may be sparse—a letter grade, a check mark, a "Great job!" at the top of the paper with no specifics—or perhaps many marks for spelling, grammar, and punctuation errors but nothing on content. Sometimes students are sent to a writing center on campus, but they often perceive this assignment as a punitive measure rather than an instructional support. Even professors who are prolific writers do not usually teach students how to write confidently, focusing instead on the ideas in their own writing. So, once again, how does one gain confidence in writing?

The answer lies in the task itself. As with any other occupation, we develop confidence in writing by writing—by engaging fully in the process. This chapter provides some suggestions to assist you in getting past the obstacles you may be facing in writing. Some suggestions may resonate with you; others you may not find helpful. Read them anyway, and reflect on them.

> As with any other occupation, we develop confidence in writing by writing—by engaging fully in the process.

Take a Writing Course

Rather than waiting for confidence to materialize out of nowhere, consider sending yourself to the writing center on campus or to an adult education center that offers a course on the process of writing. A writing center or course will confirm what you already know about writing and reiterate the following process (Scheft, 2009): Start with brainstorming, which includes reading, researching, discussing, and thinking about the topic. Write the first draft, which is just that—a draft—meaning it doesn't have to be perfect. Then get feedback from a fellow student, instructor, or trusted friend; the feedback needs to be specific to be helpful.

Next, revise the paper on the basis of the feedback—an essential part of an effective writing process. But you're not done yet. Get more feedback on your revision, and then, if necessary, continue the process until you have successfully completed the paper and can move on to handing it in or submitting it for publication. Remember that publishing is competitive and that even the most seasoned author has received more than one rejection letter. Do not consider a rejected manuscript to be a reflection on you personally; rather, consider it feedback on the degree of match between your paper and the scope of the publication you submitted to.

Say Yes to Opportunity

Life presents us with opportunities daily. Within occupational therapy, numerous opportunities appear, often when we least expect them. I have found that saying yes to opportunities has led to career success. I learn from opportunities, I have been empowered by them, and I have gained colleagues by agreeing to participate when asked. I have often been accused of not being able to say no, but the reality is that I have gained far more from saying yes than I would have by turning down opportunities. When I was asked to edit my first book, my initial response was "Why me?" But I realized that an incredible opportunity was being presented, and I took advantage of all the help that was offered to me.

Believe in Yourself

When children are growing up, they usually are encouraged, nurtured, and molded by their parents and by extended family members; teachers; caregivers; friends; mentors; and even heroes in books, television, and movies. Ideally, those early developmental experiences build a sense of self-confidence that translates into a can-do attitude and a source of internal motivation.

The time comes, however, when you have to rely on yourself. You have to be your own best friend and advocate. As you begin to develop a social network, it is important to look for people to support you and believe in you and your abilities.

Make Discipline a Habit

Psychology professor Robert Boice (1990) has written extensively about the discipline academic faculty need if they are to develop regular writing habits. It is easy to procrastinate; so many things are more interesting than the blank computer screen (see Chapter 8, this volume).

Boice (1990) described what he called *bingeing:* a pattern of writing only when up against a deadline or during a break from classes. Some academics advocate taking one day a week or even a sabbatical to write. But Boice and advocates like Belcher (2009) recommend writing daily to build the confidence that comes from a disciplined habit. Blocking out 15 minutes a day for writing will give it equal importance to any assignment, appointment, or class and help make it happen.

The creators of the occupational therapy profession wrote about *habit training,* a concept that continues to be important as a major theoretical construct. Occupational therapy practitioners develop habits in clients by teaching them to repeat tasks in a routine manner. Start a habit of writing, and reap the benefits throughout your career.

Schedule your 15 minutes at a time when you are most alert and your energy peaks. The environmental context is equally important: You will not be productive if your back is hurting because you are slumped in an uncomfortable chair, if you're developing a headache from eye strain related to inadequate lighting, or if the noise from your children playing is distracting. Select a place to write that supports your best effort and attention, and be sure the lighting and temperature are comfortable, resources are handy, and distractions are at a minimum.

Write About Yourself

You are the one who has something to say, so you need to write about your own experiences. Sometimes students get into the habit of writing in the third person which results in a sterile and emotionless piece of writing (but is often required of writing for the scholarly, technical, and medical professions). Good practice is to write daily journal entries not about what you did, but about how you felt about what you did. Write about whatever feelings, emotions, or thoughts you're experiencing, and if on rereading your writing seems superficial, rewrite and go deeper.

Writing in a journal about personal experiences leads to deep learning in which emotions may be raw and uncomfortable. But for occupational therapists to use ourselves with our clients therapeutically and to work with our colleagues, being mindful of our emotions is a critical skill. We can't be in touch with ourselves if we don't take the time to know ourselves. In addition to the deep learning that occurs, health outcomes have been linked to writing therapeutically (Pennebaker, 1997a, 1997b). If you can't think of anything to write, then write about your resistance to writing.

Know Why You Are Writing

Writing is a highly rewarding activity for anyone, and keeping an eye on these rewards can build your confidence. For health care professionals, writing is a way to advance the profession. Why do we pick up a journal and read an article? We read because we want to learn about something. Publishing is a powerful vehicle for sharing our knowledge and insights with others: "[Writing] provides the opportunity for sharing knowledge, skills and experiences with peers, which may ultimately lead to a change in clinical practice" (Happell, 2008, p. 35).

More occupational therapists are returning to school to complete advanced degrees, which generally involves disseminating the results of their studies and research (see Chapter 9 in this volume). Publication increases the evidence base for our profession, ultimately improving the care we provide to our clients. For those striving to enter academic positions, having a list of publications is a requirement for success. Writing articles brings recognition for one's knowledge and skills and leads to increased professional visibility. In addition, publishing may lead to promotion or career advancement.

Find a Mentor, Be a Mentor

A mentor is a guide for a journey. Professor Laurent Daloz (1999) wrote,

> Like guides, we walk ahead of our students, at times beside them, and at times we follow their lead. In sensing where to walk lies our art. For as we support [them] in their struggle, challenge them towards their best, and cast light on their path ahead, we do so in the name of respect for their potential and our care for their growth. (p. 244)

Having a mentor is an incredibly powerful vehicle for personal and professional growth. Wherever you are in your career, you can benefit from both having a mentor and being a mentor. Even if you are a student, you can still mentor another—a friend or acquaintance who wants to be an occupational therapy practitioner, a client who looks up to you for your ability to achieve your goals, or a younger sibling who observes the difference you are making in other peoples' lives.

Even seasoned occupational therapy practitioners can benefit from finding a mentor and working on some professional goals (see Gilfoyle, Grady, & Nielson, 2011). Throughout my career, others have been willing to serve as a mentor to me when I was facing a new challenge.

Wherever you are in your career, you can benefit from both having a mentor and being a mentor.

All you have to do is ask. Find someone who has done something you would like to do, or has worked with a similar patient population, or has written something that inspires you. Write or call that person and ask him or her to mentor you, but be certain to have some specific goals you want to work on. If you're using the mentor to help you with your writing, make sure you trust this person to give you honest feedback.

Own Your Creativity

Writing is a creative process, and the finished product is a work of art. We all have creativity, sometimes buried deep within us. In a drawing class I took as an undergraduate, the instructor told the students that we all had an innate ability to draw. He said that being told not to draw on the walls and being given coloring books and told to color within the lines stifled this creativity. I remember not wanting to take this course because I believed I could not draw, which I stated frequently in class. The instructor was patient, telling students that drawing was about observing. So he asked us to draw an object like a wristwatch over and over again. The feedback was always the same: "Look at the watch. Now look at your drawing of the watch. Do they look the same? No? Then change it so it looks like the watch." I was amazed how my drawings improved over the course of the semester without my learning any art techniques, just through repeated observations.

Owning your creativity means knowing that you can write: You've been doing it your entire life. You have life experiences and something valuable to say. The way you say it is a manifestation of your creative side.

Be Mindful in Silence

Today's world is not conducive to discipline in writing. We are rarely silent, and sounds from our environment bombard us continuously. To be successful at writing, turn down the volume on environmental noise. Find time for silence so that you can hear your thoughts: These are the ideas that you will put on paper for your finished product.

For the past 10 years, I have been learning about mindfulness and the various interventions that come out of this ancient practice (Kabat-Zinn, 1990). My first course was a 5-day silent retreat. "Silence—for 5 days—are you kidding?" I said to myself. Even my children said to me, "Mom, how are you going to be able to not talk for 5 whole days?" But in silence comes clarity of thought, an unburdening of chatter that clogs the creative mind, and an ability to engage with life as it is in the present moment.

One doesn't have to go on a retreat to learn the gift of silence and its benefits. Set aside 20 minutes a day to spend in silence meditating, praying, or being in nature. The investment of this small amount of time will give you more energy and clarity and help you move more purposefully through your days. You might want to schedule your daily writing time after this period of silence; you'll notice how much more productive you are when your mind isn't jumping from topic to topic like a monkey swinging on branches.

Stop Multitasking!

Our lives are so busy, and we have convinced ourselves that the only way we can get though our to-do list is to multitask: rushing through our list two and even three items at a time to get it all done.

Recent research on the brain has demonstrated that the brain can process only one thing at a time (Abate, 2008; Charron & Koechlin, 2010; Rosen, 2008). When we multitask, we essentially divide our attention to each item in half. When you sit down to write, writing needs to be the only task at hand: The cell phone is out of sight and sound range, the computer is not beeping every time an e-mail message is delivered, and the music you love to sing or hum to is turned off. You may be protesting at this point, "But I *can* do two things at once!" Maybe you can, but can you do them well? Maybe you can write better and faster when there are no distractions and the only task at hand for the next 15 minutes is writing. Try it as an experiment, if for no other reason. You might be pleasantly surprised.

See the Glass as Half-Full, Not Half-Empty

There is power in positive thinking, and it's not all in your head. When we believe we can do something, we can. Remember the book *The Little Engine That Could*? The engine believed he could get up the steep hill, and he succeeded. Similarly, one who expects not to succeed frequently doesn't.

The field of neurolinguistic programming (NLP) looks at language patterns and what they reveal about a person's attention. During my NLP practitioner training, I learned how to break a 1-in.-thick wooden board with my bare hand, and it is a story I often tell my students to illustrate the power of positive thinking. By using a variety of techniques aimed at telling myself that my hand could break through the board like butter, I was able to break it in half. Viewing a glass as half-full or half-empty is not necessarily innate; it can be learned. If you find that you are viewing the glass as half-empty and are not satisfied with how this way of thinking affects your life, consider reading psychologist Martin Seligman's (1998) excellent book *Learned Optimism: How to Change Your Mind and Your Life.*

Don't Wait to Publish

All too often, I have heard students and occupational therapy practitioners say they will publish someday, when they are accomplished or when they have "arrived." One of my earliest career goals was to write a book after I had been an occupational therapist for 5 years, but I didn't write my first book until after my 30th year as an occupational therapist! I didn't need to wait so long.

If you're a student, you are making discoveries in your studies and research right now. Seriously consider submitting your thesis or dissertation or capstone project to a journal (but closely follow the journal's author guidelines for submission). Even if your work isn't accepted, you will get feedback from the editors on ways to improve it, and if it is selected for publication, the thrill of seeing your name in print will be a powerful motivator for the rest of your writing career. You don't have to be the sole author; a faculty member who supervised your research can collaborate in the writing and be listed as an author.

Inspire or Motivate Others

All writers experience times when writing is difficult and can benefit from encouragement by others. You can be the motivator or inspiration for someone else. Share your writing experiences with others, and

> Seriously consider submitting your thesis or dissertation or capstone project to a journal (but closely follow the journal's author guidelines for submission).

you might find that you both benefit. Journal clubs, in which clinicians get together regularly to read and discuss articles, have become very popular. Why not start a writing club? Gather a group of peers, and meet regularly to discuss writing and give one another feedback. Have members read their writing out loud; it often allows one to hear errors that one missed on paper.

Take Up the Challenge

You want to write, and you can. I challenge you to continue writing at whatever stage you find yourself—Murray and Newton (2008) suggest taking a writing course to increase skills and self-confidence. You can also find a mentor who can coach you and give you feedback, or work with a group of colleagues to improve your writing. The occupational therapy profession needs your talents as a clinician but also as a contributor to the body of literature. Only with the knowledge passed on by its practitioners will the profession continue to flourish into our centennial year and beyond. Unruh (2007) summed up our professional mandate well:

> Writing for publication can be a gratifying and professional experience. Without publication, research and practice have limited influence on building knowledge. As our work is made available for dissemination, discussion and debate, occupational therapy and occupational science grow, mature, and influence other health professionals and researchers. (p. 61)

REFERENCES

Abate, C. (2008, Fall). You say multitasking like it's a good thing. *Thought and Action* (The National Education Higher Education Journal), pp. 7–13.

Belcher, W. L. (2009). Reflections on ten years of teaching writing for publication to graduate students and junior faculty. *Journal of Scholarly Publishing, 40*, 184–199. doi: 10:3138/jsp.40.2.184

Boice, R. (1990). *Professors as writers: A self-help guide to productive writing.* Stillwater, OK: New Forums Press.

Charron, S., & Koechlin, E. (2010). Divided representation of concurrent goals in the human frontal lobes. *Science, 328*(5976), 360–363.

Daloz, L. (1999). *Mentor: Guiding the journey of adult learners.* San Francisco: Jossey-Bass.

Gilfoyle, E., Grady, A., & Nielson, C. (2011). *Mentoring leaders: The power of storytelling for building leadership in health care and education*. Bethesda, MD: AOTA Press.

Happell, B. (2008). Writing for publication: A practical guide. *Nursing Standard, 22*(28), 35–40.

Kabat-Zinn, J. (1990). *Full catastrophe living: Using the wisdom of your body and mind to face stress, pain, and illness*. New York: Delta/Bantam Dell/Random House.

Murray, R., & Newton, M. (2008). Facilitating writing for publication. *Physiotherapy, 94*, 29–34.

Pennebaker, J. (1997a). *Opening up: The healing power of expressing emotions*. New York: Guilford.

Pennebaker, J. (1997b). Writing about emotional experiences as a therapeutic process. *Psychological Science, 8*, 162–166.

Plath, S. (1982). *The journals of Sylvia Plath*. New York: Doubleday.

Rosen, C. (2008, Spring). The myth of multitasking. *The New Atlantis*, pp. 105–110.

Scheft, T. (2009). *Inspiring student writers: Strategies and examples for teachers*. Charlotte, NC: Information Age.

Seligman, M. (1998). *Learned optimism: How to change your mind and your life*. New York: Free Press.

Unruh, A. (2007). Reflections on . . . writing for successful publication. *Canadian Journal of Occupational Therapy, 74*, 61–68.

2

Roles, Rituals, and Habits of a Writer

ELIZABETH CARA, PhD, OTR/L, MFT

This . . . is about writing. It is also about using writing as your practice, as a way to help you penetrate your life and become sane. What is said here about writing can be applied to running, painting, anything you love and have chosen to work with in your life.

—NATALIE GOLDBERG (1986, P. 3)

Being a writer is not a usual place for an occupational therapist or for an academic in an allied health field. We are usually more focused on research or practice, on what interventions work. Occupational therapists often focus on people's stories, however, and the meaning revealed in them. Ironies, it seems, are an essential part of the writing process; sometimes writing takes us to new places and new spaces within ourselves. In writing *psychobiography*—a story about another person—I found my passion, learned about myself, and came to know myself in a new way.

I have not always practiced writing or considered myself a writer. My writing evolved in many forms over many years and many careers. This chapter is the story of my writing practices and how I became a writer. It is also the story of how I came to choose what I write, particularly my experience in writing about Dian Fossey (Cara, 2007a), who was a primatologist and occupational therapist made famous through the book and movie

Gorillas in the Mist (Apted & Phelan, 1988; Fossey, 1983). I invite you to learn about my writing process and to develop a writing practice as a meaningful occupation encompassing habits, routines, roles, rituals, interests, contexts, and environments, just as I have. I hope that my story will inspire you to become the writer you were meant to be, for that one project or for a lifetime.

Roles

Writing emerged out of the many roles I have engaged in, mostly tied to my career. I graduated with a BA in history. My course work required me to write historical papers for each of my classes. After receiving my degree, I went back to school to become an occupational therapist. My first job, in mental health, was at a large psychiatric hospital with many other therapists; I wrote evaluation reports, treatment plans, and progress notes and actually enjoyed that creative process. In that setting, we were given the opportunity to develop groups. I developed a group focused on a need that I recognized for women who were depressed and gave it a catchy title—the Self-Sufficiency Group for Women. It was very successful and was recognized as such by my colleagues. I was encouraged to share the group concept with mental health occupational therapists. Hence, I wrote a proposal, which was accepted, for a presentation at the national conference.

I presented before a large audience (Cara, 1977), and I realized that presenting to an audience was motivating for me. I liked putting together material that made sense, and I enjoyed sharing it. I also came to understand that I liked the give-and-take and excitement of a presentation—not unlike running groups in mental health—and of having the stage and sharing my thoughts with people who listened. The (mostly) positive attention my presentation afforded was satisfying, and I felt encouraged.

I had gravitated to mental health because it was exciting, unpredictable, and different every day, and it allowed me to use my creativity daily. I gravitated toward group treatment because it also had the same qualities of difference, excitement, and unpredictability, with one additional quality: leading. Groups allowed me to "be on stage"—to act, so to speak—and I loved that. In a group process, I was able to help people tell their story and have a stage for themselves, and I found that equally rewarding.

It is not surprising that I became a professor, because teaching a class has aspects similar to leading groups and providing mental health treatment. Within my role of worker, I first chose what to write, presentations, on the basis of my work in groups and my joy in being able to act and direct and being (somewhat) a focus of attention, but in a process that allowed me to be a catalyst for others' thoughts. Thus, my desire to share successful treatment with colleagues was my initial motivation for writing.

After working in mental health for a decade, I decided to learn more about people and mental health and to deepen my professional skills for doing and facilitating storytelling. I set a goal of becoming a psychotherapist and obtained my master's degree in clinical psychology. For my degree, I had to write a master's thesis. Writing a thesis was unlike writing the historical papers of my undergraduate work; the thesis was more formal and scientific, with a structured format to follow and research to be accomplished. However, writing a thesis was not unlike writing as a clinician, although as a clinician I wrote more briefly.

In 1990 I began teaching at San José State University and committed to being an educator. Therefore, I obtained a doctoral degree in my field, clinical psychology. For my doctorate I had to write a dissertation, and in academia I have to conduct and write up research. Thus, much of what I have to write is dictated by my career. As a professor, I am expected to publish my research and to write textbooks, presentations, and grant proposals—what I call *technical writing* in that there are specific formats to follow. Technical writing is nonfiction, but it is very different nonfiction than psychobiography.

Although I would not have said this when I first published a textbook (Cara & MacRae, 1998), textbooks are probably the most creative of all the writing I have mentioned so far. They require editors to create their own format for the book and chapters. Research, presentations, and grant proposals do not allow for much deviation from format, and any deviation (especially in quantitative research) is quickly deleted or edited out. Textbooks allow more leeway.

> **Research, presentations, and grant proposals do not allow for much deviation from format, and any deviation (especially in quantitative research) is quickly deleted or edited out. Textbooks allow more leeway.**

The impetus for writing psychobiography, my ultimate passion in writing, was similar to my motivation for writing research studies, presentations, grant proposals, and textbooks in occupational therapy: to share with my occupational therapy colleagues and the profession what I thought was missing. In so doing, I am gaining a little fame from my work. Coming to this realization about this part of myself—that I enjoy the roles of actor and director—developed through the process of writing. Truthfully, it was not until I began thinking about and writing this chapter that I learned so surely about this space in myself.

This process of realization through many forms of writing for my careers in occupational therapy is what I call *occupational coherence* (Cara, 2007a). Although the forms and roles were seemingly different, they all contributed to my identity as a writer. *Occupational coherence* is "a work life consisting of occupations that are imbued with value and meaning which convey and sustain a cohesive identity throughout a person's life" (p. 150). All of these endeavors produced a product that brought me deep satisfaction. They also signified that I could convey some part of myself to others in multiple forums, and I was rewarded by a sense of joy when doing so. They helped maintain my career and earned money, but they also included the sense of play that reading and learning have always given me, and I enjoyed a true recreational value by putting the pieces together and acting in these established roles.

So my roles as clinician, group leader, and professor enabled me to engage in the occupation of writing. But my temperament and personality also came through in my enjoyment of being an actor and director of the presentations or groups or the author of texts. In the occupational process of writing, I became a writer and learned about personality aspects that were perhaps waiting to be manifested in my life.

Temperament and Interests

Some of the joy I experience from presenting and writing relates directly to my temperament and personality and can be explained in terms of client factors, specifically global mental functions, as defined in the *Occupational Therapy Practice Framework: Domain and Process* (American Occupational Therapy Association [AOTA], 2008). In addition, my experience of self and time and my emotional coping and regulation are specific mental functions in *Framework* terminology. My beliefs and values influence me; my interests influence why and what I write.

Like any writer, I love to read. Reading can be described in different ways using the *Framework*: Reading is

- An area of occupation, education, and leisure and work
- A client factor, value, and mental function
- A cognitive performance skill
- A performance pattern that is a habit
- Performed in a cultural and virtual context.

Reading has always transported me to other places and shown me how individuals and groups of people think and act. I have simply taken pleasure in reading, and it has always been a joy. Even as a child, I often picked up anything around me to read, even my dad's *U.S. News & World Report* or *Business Week*. Reading has always been a solace to me when I experienced difficult life events or family stress. Reading not only transported me or satisfied my interests but also illustrated how others organize words. Thus, reading was a natural way of sampling how others write.

As Miller and Paola (2005) acknowledged, "There's no getting around it: Reading and writing go hand in hand" (p. 175). Thus, my roles as professor, occupational therapy clinician in mental health, marriage and family counselor, and graduate student combined to organize me as a writer. My personality and temperament added to my motivation to write and present, and my interests born originally of my background of being attuned to people also led me to write about people and the places my mind has traveled to through my reading.

As long as I can remember, I have always tried to make sense of historical events and the past. I think some of the difficulties and family events I experienced when I was young (e.g., deaths, divorces, blended families, mental health issues) predisposed me to be very attuned to other people and how others acted the way they did. Therefore, it was almost inevitable that I became interested in psychobiography. It was a natural evolution to become interested in writing people's lives, just as I was interested in healing people in the mental health field and in educating people in the academic field.

Attraction to Psychobiography

When I became an occupational therapist in 1975, I had never heard of Dian Fossey, the primatologist who saved the great apes from extinction. Reading about Fossey was easy. There is plenty written about her because she was a controversial figure who accomplished unusual feats. I read everything she wrote, including her *National Geographic* articles (Fossey, 1970, 1971) and her book *Gorillas in the Mist* (Fossey, 1983).

As a student of writing, I read books about writing (my favorite ones are quoted throughout this chapter). As a psychobiographer, I read about the craft of psychobiography and biography writing (Carlson, 1988; Elms, 1994, 2005; McAdams, 1988, 2005; Runyan, 1982, 1988, 2005; Young-Bruehl, 1998). I followed the advice I heard on imitation and read what I considered to be the best psychobiographies (Breslin, 1993; Elms, 1994; Young-Bruehl, 1988). My joy in reading easily translated to a habit of researching psychobiographies. Now I am writing a book about Fossey! And I am already planning another psychobiography, about the American artist Georgia O'Keeffe.

Psychobiography is a nonfiction form of narrative writing that tells the life story of another person, often one who is no longer living. It is a biography or life history of a person, and what makes it a "psycho" biography is that I make interpretations about Fossey's motivations and about how her personality, background, and environment may have prompted her to do what she did and to act the way she acted. My interpretations are grounded in reflexivity and facts that gestate over time. That is, they are not based on speculation.

For example, speculation would amount to reading about a person and then making a quick judgment without a reasoning process based on what you just read. It is as if it would be the first thought that came to your mind. A psychobiographical interpretation is based on critical analysis or reasoning—checking your interpretations with other experts, material synthesized from documents, and interviews with others who knew the person or autobiographical statements. A psychobiography thus has coherence and credibility and evidence that is not present in a speculation.

Writing psychobiography is an occupational process. It is particularly surprising that I write about Fossey because she immersed herself in the lives of nonhuman primates, and I had never been interested in books about animals, even as a kid. I was acutely intrigued by Fossey's passions, though, so I wrote about her not because of an interest in primatology or animals but because she was an occupational therapist who graduated from San José State, the program in which I teach, and was a person who did extraordinary things. Writings about her vary greatly, from supportive to highly critical (Hayes, 1990; Mowat, 1987; Shoumatoff, 1986; Torgovnick, 1997; Villagran, 1988; Weber & Vedder, 2001), but I uncovered a key flaw in these writings that disturbed me: Occupational therapy was neither explained nor even mentioned in more than one sentence.

In fact, the profession was often disregarded or denigrated. The movie about her, *Gorillas in the Mist,* did not even recognize her as an occupational therapist! I thought to myself, "This just is not right." My sense of injustice, violation of values, and resulting anger propelled me to investigate further and set the record straight. Indeed, my anger motivated me to find and write the "other" story that I thought surely must be there. Thus, my passion moved me to write (and continues to do so). As Goldberg (1986) explained, "Your main obsessions have power; they are what you will come back to in your writing over and over again. And you'll create new stories around them" (p. 38).

The more I researched and wrote, the more the people in my life, in my writing group and others, urged me to write a book. After publishing papers on Fossey (Cara, 2007a, 2007b) and conducting more years of research, I presented a version of my book proposal to my psychobiography group.[1] Some group members agreed that I should lead with Fossey's career in occupational therapy because I was the only person who understood that very important part of her life. But I was angry about that piece of her life being left out, and I believed that I had to set aside my anger about the denigration and minimization of Fossey's first profession. I believed that an author was required to be neutral to write well.

But I've come to see this belief as the academic tone intruding and limiting my full exploration of the psychobiographical method of writing. One reviewer surprised me when she said, "You are so angry about this. Every time you present, you are so annoyed that people do not know about occupational therapy and about her career before she went to Africa; you should

---

[1]This group was originally called the San Francisco Bay Area Psychobiography *Study Group and was supported by the Townsend Center* of the University of California at Berkeley.

keep that anger when you write!" My fellow group members wholeheartedly agreed, and from that time forward I felt freed to acknowledge how I felt and to write from my heart.

This freedom and heartfelt writing came only, and I do mean only, because I surrounded myself with writers and a group of like-minded people dedicated to writing and to improving their writing. Each of us in the group agrees that writers, especially psychobiographers, must rigorously examine themselves constantly and consistently in relationship to what they write. We practice that habit in all of our meetings and presentations and critiques. I thought, perhaps I *am* the only person who has the occupational therapy perspective and who is angry, but tempered enough, to set the story straight. I can and want (and need?) to do this.

Habits

Over the years, I've cultivated several habits that facilitate my occupation of writing: working with other writers, imitating other writers, presenting my work for critique and support, meeting deadlines, continually revising and editing, learning everything I can about my subject, and using notebooks.

WORKING WITH OTHER WRITERS

> Writers need feedback. The myth of writers as loners who follow their vision and remain true to their inner muse, bucking rather than embracing outside help, is very much a myth. (Miller & Paola, 2005, p. 162)

> Anything we fully do is an alone journey. . . . You are alone when you write a book. . . . You can't expect anyone to match the intensity of your emotions or to completely understand what you went through. (Goldberg, 1986, p. 169)

Writing is a habit, a practice, and a journey at once solitary and social. I have felt simultaneously alone in the solitary act of writing down my thoughts and emotions and supported by outside help from the members of my writing group. Most of our work was psychobiographical, but some members expanded into memoirs and other nonfiction or tried out new genres or forms of expression. In this group, I practiced the habits of reading and evaluating material similar to what I wrote, critically analyzing different styles and forms, and working intimately with other writers to achieve our goals.

IMITATING OTHER WRITERS

The group also afforded me an opportunity that teachers of writing often stress—the opportunity to imitate other writers. I followed the advice of Zinsser (2006): "Never hesitate to imitate another writer. Imitation is part of the creative process for anyone learning an art or a craft" (p. 235). I was able to read an abundance of papers over many years; as a professor I read research papers to prepare for my classes, as a clinician I kept up with the latest developments in the field, and in my writing group we read one another's work and discussed what constitutes good or bad writing. I was able to take the good and use the best styles while gaining some ideas about how not to write.

PRESENTING MY WORK FOR CRITIQUE AND SUPPORT

In the group I also practiced another habit of a writer, presenting my work to others for critique and support. When I present my work, I invite others to critique and comment on my writing style and process, both conscious and unconscious. Their critiques and the discussions that follow, although difficult to receive sometimes—it is difficult to place myself back in the role of novice—have been invaluable to me. The process has moved my writing forward, and I have become a better writer. Sharing my work with others is not just about critique; many people have supported and encouraged me and helped with my reflection process. A supportive group or individual does not mean one who always agrees with you but rather one who is invested in seeing that you learn to write well and delve further into your values and purpose in writing. So an attitude of acceptance toward criticism is important in improving your writing. For me, the group and the constant evaluating atmosphere of academia have helped me realize that critique and evaluation, when motivated by caring, really help a writer improve.

MEETING DEADLINES

Being in a writing group also motivated me to set deadlines for completing writing projects. Each member of the writing group not only wrote but also prepared presentations about their work for analysis; therefore,

> An attitude of acceptance toward criticism is important in improving your writing.

when I made a commitment to present, I had to do it. The need to meet a deadline is very important to motivate me to actually, physically, sit down and write.

CONTINUALLY REVISING AND EDITING

One of the habits most crucial to making me a better writer was to constantly revise (writing new versions of the paper over time so that sometimes it does not look at all like the original) and edit (go through the paper line by line to make spelling or grammatical changes or looking for better phrasing). Some authors write seven or more drafts of a work. Goldberg (1986) encouraged writers to

> See revision as "envisioning again." If there are areas in your work where there is a blur or vagueness, you can simply see the picture again and add the details that will bring your work closer to your mind's picture. (p. 165)

Along with the habit of rewriting, a writer must edit, edit, edit, and edit again. The advice I've been given (and have taken) is to be ruthless in eliminating anything that is not absolutely crucial to the understanding of a sentence.

I tend to be a broad and expansive thinker. Therefore, when I write I include many ideas. I am not the type of writer who carefully follows one idea to conclusion. One of my group members exclaimed, when I presented my first paper on Dian Fossey, "You have 13 different papers in this one!" I've grown used to this feedback and accept it as positive and useful critique. In fact, instead of being thwarted by these many papers hiding in one, I edited the original paper (at least 10 times over many years), and it morphed into two published papers—one about Fossey (Cara, 2007a) and the other on how to write psycho-biographies (Cara, 2007b)—and even a proposal for an edited book about Fossey.

LEARNING EVERYTHING I CAN ABOUT MY SUBJECT

When I undertake an endeavor or occupational performance, I do not "just do it." One important habit I have is to learn everything I can about what I am doing. This has always been true, whether I am cooking, engaging in athletic pursuits, going to a museum, or reading fiction and nonfiction. I have always and consistently read and learned as much as possible about it. Thus, as I write, I read how-to books on writing skills and books about others' personal narratives and the reasons that propel them to write. Although the habit of reading has given me insights into how to do or perform my own writing and has always helped my occupational performance, I also believe that "the only correct way to write is the way that works for you" (Miller & Paola, 2005, p. 153) and that "every writer must follow the path that feels most comfortable" (Zinsser, 2006, p. 99).

USING NOTEBOOKS

Another habit that supports me in writing is to carry notebooks with me wherever I go (a tablet such as the iPad might work as well for those writers who prefer to work online). I used to underline important passages in books or mark them with sticky notes; now, I have modified that habit to taking notes and copying quotes with citations into small notebooks (one could perhaps use the highlighting feature in e-book apps).

Carrying notebooks is easy for me because I love them, and I buy special notebooks from museums or art stores or for specific books that I read. For writing, I carry small notebooks with southwestern designs that I purchased in Santa Fe, New Mexico, a place I travel to often and that has magical and memorable aspects. At home I use small yellow tablets. My system, perhaps elevated to ritual by now, is to label my notes in the margins as I take them. For example, about Fossey, some labels were *Africa, illnesses, social, gorillas and play, her statements,* and *motivations.* All of my notes on Fossey are in inexpensive notebooks that fit nicely between the pages of whatever book I may be reading—for ease of carrying. Although I eventually started taking notes with my computer, I never really became comfortable with that or with bibliographic programs. So I still use notebooks.

Some writers use the same pen or special pens when they write or take notes. I do not have a special pen, but I always use the same brand, and I have these pens in every purse, briefcase, backpack, and desk that I might use when writing. Occasionally, I write passages in yellow tablets with a pencil because it is easier to erase and edit as I write. Erasing as I go helps curb my tendency to keep every word because I think that they are so important; pencil allows me to edit out sooner what is superfluous or could be better stated.

Rituals

For me, rituals around writing are all about ways to initiate writing. Goldberg (1986) got it right when she said, "It is important to have a way worked out to begin your writing; otherwise, washing the dishes becomes the most important thing on earth—anything that will divert you from writing" (p. 24). The most important things on earth as I thought about sitting down to write were shopping for new clothes or seeing the latest art exhibit. Just as I told myself I would write, I decided right then that everything in my closet was old and I needed new clothes.

One incongruous aspect of Fossey's life in the jungle observing gorillas, with all the dirt and mess that entailed, was that she had been a debutante known by everyone for her way with accessorizing her clothing and look. Somehow, as I began to write I thought that my obsession with clothes at that moment was appropriate for Fossey research. But the ritual that finally got me to actually do the writing was going to a café. Maybe at home I could easily divert myself, but going to a café was a joy where words often flowed. Working in a café, as so many authors and artists had done before me, meant that maybe I truly was a writer. Also, cafés are great places to be solitary but also to be surrounded by familiar people.

Once I'm settled at a table, another part of my ritual for getting started is to allow myself to be awkward rather than expecting a smooth start, knowing that later I can edit or revise. In addition, Goldberg (1986) noted that there is no perfect atmosphere, notebook, pen, or desk for writing, so I've trained myself to be flexible by writing under different circumstances and in different places. Thus, I have written about Fossey in many places other than cafés—on buses, subways, and trains and in cars—although cafés remain the best place for me to write.

Client Factors

Client factors are "specific abilities, characteristics, or beliefs that reside within [a person that] may affect performance in areas of occupation" (AOTA, 2008, p. 630)—writing, in my case. These factors include values, beliefs, spirituality, and body functions, including cognition and mental health.

My values, then—especially my commitment to justice—propelled me to write/right the story of Dian Fossey. Although as a psychobiographer I desired to be as honest as possible when writing about her qualities, both positive and negative, I just did not think it was right that she was denigrated in print as much as she was. I sought out a fuller picture of her and her work. In this endeavor I obviously believed that there was a fuller story to be told and that it should be told by someone who knew about her earlier life and was willing to be rigorously honest with herself in telling the story. I do not necessarily consider myself a spiritual person, but some may consider a quest to uncover and tell the truth as honestly as they know it simultaneously to be a mindful and a spiritual quest.

The very act of writing requires certain mental functions. For example, in writing about Fossey, although at times it seemed difficult to put words to a page in an articulate way, I had to possess the higher-level cognitive functions of insight, attention, and awareness. In each single act of writing, one displays cognitive flexibility, memory, and attention.

To write, one has to experience oneself in time. Thus, although I may not always feel it, I have to have some coherent sense of self and enough self-esteem to believe I can write. When I began writing psychobiography I was not sure that I could write as well as my colleagues, but I did think enough of myself to give it a try. I did not think of myself as a writer, but in the process of writing I did come to identify myself as a writer, first of research papers, now of books. I lived the occupational therapy belief in doing and becoming (Fidler & Fidler, 1978).

The most important mental function for me, and I think for everyone who writes, is emotional. To write, one experiences ups and downs, triumphs and frustrations. I believe myself to be awful sometimes and absolutely destitute of words or sentences that sound even halfway articulate. Therefore, coping and behavioral regulation are essential. I experience the triumphs and frustrations of writing particularly when I write psychobiography. I have much passion and esteem (as well as time, years, and energy) invested in writing about Fossey and other subjects close to my heart; therefore, how I cope with those valleys of inarticulation is particularly important to keep me motivated and tenacious.

> To write, one experiences ups and downs, triumphs and frustrations. . . . Therefore, coping and behavioral regulation are essential.

As Miller and Paola (2005) stated, "Do whatever it takes to refill the well" (p. 172). My ability to stick with it derives from my personality and temperament, partly, but also from talking positively to myself and being supported by others. Hearing my writing group friends' personal stories about their struggles normalizes my own struggles. But I also often tell myself, "Oh, this impasse is part of the typical nature of writing; I will experience these struggles in the process."

Reading about others who have overcome catastrophic life events also lightens my troubles. Instead of telling myself that my struggles are insignificant or that life seems insurmountable, I tell myself, "These people overcame huge, seemingly impossible events to continue living and loving. Therefore, I can easily overcome this small, noncatastrophic event of not writing well right now."

I often talk to myself as a way of continuing when writing is not going so well. For example, I tell myself, "I will just write a half-page today" or "I'll sleep on this and wake up with some new ideas." Sometimes, when I'm spiraling into a downward cycle of thinking that I have no business writing, I simply shout to myself, *"Stop it!"* Sometimes I take a walk or go have a caffe latte (if it's the morning) or green tea latte (if it's the afternoon), a ritual I've become known for and have practiced since the 1970s. Or I may just change the scenery or watch football. At other times, I stop what I am doing and carry on some other part of writing, whether editing or reviewing what I have already written or looking up citations. I may decide that it is best to do some other work and not write for that period or day because I am not in an emotional place to write. At these times, I "refill the well" by walking, hiking or swimming, going to the gym or to a museum, reading *O* magazine or *Art News,* or calling a friend.

Contexts and Environments

I use the temporal and virtual contexts, as well as the physical (natural or constructed) and social environment, to enable my participation in the occupation of writing (AOTA, 2008).

TIME

Although I have a belief that I should get up early in the morning and write for 4 hours (on the days I do not teach), I have rarely practiced that!

Instead, I get up and out of the house to a café and start the day by reading the paper. Then I do errands, sometimes work out at the gym, and then settle in to write. So my temporal pattern is to write in the early afternoon for a few hours. I usually write for about 2 hours, then take a break, and perhaps return later to writing for about an hour or two longer.

At rare times I have woken up and written early in the morning, and I still believe this is best because my thinking is clearer and sharper early in the morning and I am less distracted, so I offer this advice to fledgling writers. I motivate myself by rewarding myself after writing for a certain amount of time; sometimes the reward is simply relief that I have already written and that even if I do not write more that day, I have accomplished the task.

DEVICES

I write now with a computer (virtual context) but have not always done so. When I began writing for my career in the early 1990s, I always wrote by hand on plain tablets or paper. The physical act of writing by hand seemed to prompt me to write more freely. It took a long time for me to begin to write on a computer because typing did not give me the same free-flowing feeling. As electronic devices became more available and smaller and lighter, however, I moved to writing on a computer. When I began writing about Fossey, I had fully transitioned to writing with a computer, although I sometimes use notebooks when I have ideas and am not close to a computer. I have also been known to write on napkins!

PHYSICAL AND SOCIAL ENVIRONMENT

The physical and social environments are both crucial to my writing process. I am most comfortable when writing in a café surrounded by people and activity but not necessarily interacting with them. I am also comfortable writing at home at the same desk in the same work space, which usually is light and sunny and has a lot of windows to see outside. Fossey's story was written mostly in my home office and the patio of my favorite café. I have never written about Fossey, or anyone else, in my office at work, which is too far away from home to just pop into to write.

Although the activity in a café is usually helpful to me, the music cannot be too loud, and I do not like to wear earphones or have the sound of music coming from earphones. When I am writing in my home office, I write to soothing Renaissance music that includes ballads, often religious ballads from pilgrimages or Christian and Jewish Spain and early musical instruments such as harp, baroque guitars, conch shell, the lute, or the viola da gamba. The music also has to fit my mood; if I am in a more serious or somber mood, I listen to cello music (Pablo Casals or Yo-Yo Ma). Any other music is usually distracting for me and does not provide an environment that is conducive for writing. I've come to know this about myself and to understand what supports my goals and what impedes them.

My physical writing environment has to be organized. Having piles of folders or books strewn around makes me unable to write; any books and folders have to be arranged neatly. I also cannot write in a messy room or with too many knickknacks or clutter around me. It is important to have some of my special things around me, however, such as books that I treasure or fine art and crafts. When writing about Fossey, I have her book *Gorillas in the Mist* handy, as well as other biographies and books about Fossey, Rwanda, or Africa and about psychobiography. In addition, I have a stuffed mountain gorilla from the Dian Fossey Gorilla Foundation, given to me by two students who worked with me one semester, and other gorilla collectibles that friends have given me.

Discovering Your Process for Writing

I became a writer after many years of writing and a passion for psychobiography. A combination of roles, habits, routines, interests, values, contexts, environments, and personality traits combined to enable what I write and organize how I write. The most important motivational and supporting aspects of writing have been a writing group, writing itself, a passion to know more about people, and openness to critique. All of these aspects developed through time in a process that has been sometimes frustrating but ultimately satisfying and joyful.

To aspiring writers, I offer the advice to get to know yourself by identifying the interests, values, routines, habits, contexts, and environments that are enabling, and you will become a writer as you write. I hope that you will discover what motivates and enables your writing and will follow your passion. As I say to all of my students, if you want to learn how to write, then write, and start now!

REFERENCES

American Occupational Therapy Association. (2008). Occupational therapy practice framework: Domain and process (2nd ed.). *American Journal of Occupational Therapy, 62,* 625–683. doi:10.5014/ajot.62.6.625

Apted, M. (Director), & Phelan, A. H. (Writer). (1988). *Gorillas in the mist* [Motion picture]. United States: Universal Studios, Warner Bros.

Breslin, J. (1993). *Mark Rothko: A biography.* Chicago: University of Chicago Press.

Cara, E. (1977, April). *Coping with the Bell Jar—A self-sufficiency group for women based on a cognitive therapy approach.* Presentation at the AOTA National Conference, San Juan, Puerto Rico.

Cara, E. (2007a). An example of occupational coherence: The story of Dian Fossey, occupational therapist and primatologist. *British Journal of Occupational Therapy, 70*(4), 147–153.

Cara, E. (2007b). Psychobiography: A research method in search of a home. *British Journal of Occupational Therapy, 70*(3), 115–121.

Cara, E., & MacRae, A. (Eds.). (1998). *Psychosocial occupational therapy: A clinical practice.* Clifton Park, NY: Delmar.

Carlson, R. (1988). *Exemplary lives: The uses of psychobiography for theory development.* In D. McAdams & R. Ochberg (Eds.), *Psychobiography and life narratives* (pp. 105–138). Durham, NC: Duke University Press.

Elms, A. C. (1994). *Uncovering lives: The uneasy alliance of biography and psychology.* New York: Oxford University Press.

Elms, A. C. (2005). If the glove fits: The art of theoretical choice in psychobiography. In W. T. Schultz (Ed.), *Handbook of psychobiography* (pp. 84–103). New York: Oxford University Press.

Fidler, G., & Fidler, J. (1978). Doing and becoming. *American Journal of Occupational Therapy, 23*(5), 305–310.

Fossey, D. (1970). Making friends with mountain gorillas. *National Geographic, 137,* 48–67.

Fossey, D. (1971). More years with mountain gorillas. *National Geographic, 140,* 574–585.

Fossey, D. (1983). *Gorillas in the mist.* Boston: Houghton Mifflin.

Goldberg, N. (1986). *Writing down the bones: Freeing the writer within.* Boston: Shambhala.

Hayes, H. T. P. (1990). *The dark romance of Dian Fossey.* New York: Touchstone.

McAdams, D. P. (1988). Biography, narrative, and lives: An introduction. *Journal of Personality, 56*(1), 1–17.

McAdams, D. P. (2005). What psychobiographers might learn from personality psychology. In W. T. Schultz (Ed.), *Handbook of psychobiography* (pp. 64–83). New York: Oxford University Press.

Miller, B., & Paola, S. (2005). *Tell it slant: Writing and shaping creative nonfiction.* New York: McGraw-Hill.

Mowat, F. (1987). *Woman in the mists: The story of Dian Fossey and the mountain gorillas of Africa.* New York: Warner Books.

Runyan, W. M. (1982). *Life histories and psychobiography: Explorations in theory and method.* New York: Oxford University Press.

Runyan, W. M. (Ed.). (1988). *Psychology and historical interpretation.* New York: Oxford University Press.

Runyan, W. M. (2005). How to critically evaluate alternative explanations of life events: The case of Van Gogh's ear. In W. T. Schultz (Ed.), *Handbook of psychobiography* (pp. 96–103). New York: Oxford University Press.

Shoumatoff, A. (1986, January). The fatal obsession of Dian Fossey. *Vanity Fair,* pp. 84–90.

Torgovnick, M. (1997). *Primitive passions: Men, women and the quest for ecstasy.* New York: Knopf.

Villagran, N. (1988, September 26). Fossey's obsession. *San Jose Mercury News,* pp. 9B, 16B.

Weber, B., & Vedder, A. (2001). *In the kingdom of the gorillas: Fragile species in a dangerous land.* New York: Simon & Schuster.

Young-Bruehl, E. (1988). *Anna Freud: A biography.* New York: Simon & Schuster.

Young-Bruehl, E. (1998). *Subject to biography: Psychoanalysis, feminism, and writing women's lives.* Cambridge, MA: Harvard University Press.

Zinsser, W. (2006). *On writing well: The classic guide to writing non-fiction.* New York: HarperCollins.

Finding Your Voice and Giving It Away

SUZANNE M. PELOQUIN, PhD, OTR, FAOTA

*Nothing on earth is more gladdening than knowing we must roll up our
sleeves and move back the boundaries of the humanly possible once more.*

—ANNIE DILLARD (1989)

I s any one of the following true? You've thought about writing. Your
nature is more suited to words on paper than to debates in committees.
You savor words. Some say your ideas stand a bit off the beaten path.
Others find your thoughts intriguing. Someone has suggested that you
"write up" what you're doing. You'd like to share your strong beliefs.
A friend reads your Christmas letter and quips, "You really ought to write!"
You enjoy puns; you like phrases that are rhythmic. Or, conversely and
almost perversely, you labor over writing but love those moments when you
are taken by words to a thrilling place. If any of these scenarios rings true,
you've already flirted with the thought of writing. You're ready to more
seriously consider the questions that follow flirtation.

Two categories of questions occur to one who considers writing. The first
is, "Do I have ideas worth sharing?" followed quickly by the corollary, "Can
I share ideas in a worthwhile way?" These categorical questions transcend
grammar and composition to reach the deeper matter of voice—finding and

giving voice. Finding voice starts with finding a topic to which one can speak with either passion or authority. *Finding voice* is the "what" or subject matter of writing. *Giving voice* is using words to share the topic well; it is the "how" or style of writing. When a person weds topic and style in a deeply satisfying way, the outcome is a sense of that person's "having a voice" in writing. When a writer conveys big ideas in a winning style, that goodness of fit shapes a writer's power. Although finding and giving voice are distinct aspects of good writing, the two are inseparable. Finding voice is only half of writing. The work spent capturing and sharing ideas well calls on the other half, giving voice.

At some point in the quest for a unique voice, a person discerns writing as meaningful. This discernment is one that occupational therapists every-where can understand: A person becomes meaningfully occupied by writ-ing. Listen to author Annie Dillard (1989), who has engaged in a lifetime of writing and compared it to other occupations:

> When you write, you lay out a line of words. The line of words is a miner's pick, a woodcarver's gouge, a surgeon's probe. You wield it, and it digs a path you follow. Soon you find yourself in new territory. (p. 3)

In each of Dillard's metaphors, even as purposeful activity is described, more than purpose is implied. Mining, carving, and performing surgery are all hard work. But the promise of finding more within each adds meaning to the process: A miner's pick may hit ore. An artist's gouge may carve a treasure. A surgeon's probe may yield a cure. Engagement with writing as an occupation presses one to embrace the work for its purpose *and* its promise.

In the writing territory that Dillard describes, voice-related issues of passion and style are part of the landscape. Passion for a topic of value, mastery of style, commitment to the process, and validation of the work— these are the subjects of this chapter. My view is this: Finding and giving voice stand together as kindred occupations, the favorable outcome of which makes for a writer a "place" in writing that feels right. I believe that finding and giving voice are within reach of a new writer's grasp.

Finding Voice: A Topic Worth Sharing

When Wendy Wood (2005) first launched the column "A Firm Persuasion in Our Work" as associate editor of the *American Journal of Occupational*

Therapy (AJOT), she titled it using David Whyte's (2001) words: "To have a firm persuasion in our work—to feel that what we do is right for ourselves and good for the world at the same time—is one of the great triumphs of human existence" (p. 4). Those who find a voice in writing feel a like-minded triumph. But how does one begin that quest?

Finding a voice starts with the belief that one has something to say. Many conditions prompt writers to pick up a pen or sit at a keyboard. The choice of topic may turn on many circumstances but often comes back to passion and purpose. Occupational injustice stoked the writing of Elizabeth Townsend and Gail Whiteford (2005). Deep respect for diversity led Michael Iwama (2005) to share his Kawa (river) model. The promise of sensory integration pressed A. Jean Ayres (1963) to write. Finding topics to which one is intensely drawn is a gift. Identifying topics to which one is inclined is a step in that direction. There seems to be a continuum of a writer's interest, at the high end of which stands some hallmark idea. Yet author Julia Alvarez (2003) invoked caution when it comes to naming a writer's passion:

> I hear the cage of a definition close around me with its "subject matter," "style," or "concerns." I find that the best way to define myself is through the stories and poems that do not limit me to a simple label, a choice. Maybe it is part of my immigrant uneasiness at the question, in whatever form, "Do you have something to declare?" (p. 133)

Like Alvarez, some writers feel trapped by the notion of naming their "one" passion. Other writers recall their writing in its unfolding and name the passion. Listen to novelist Patricia Cornwell (2003):

> I have become—for reasons even I do not fully understand—a passionate student of crime. No matter how well I may do, I can never forsake the work that got me where I am—the dogged research into time of death, the slide in the lab, the slab in the morgue. (p. 155)

My passion crept in slowly. My first penchant was to learn more about patient–therapist connections. I had little experience or authority, but my desire was strong. I enrolled in a counseling program and there found ideas that meshed well with occupational therapy. I wanted to share these, so I wrote my first article as a novice practitioner. A doctoral program led to more learning. Because I still practiced occupational therapy, I had unending questions about patients, about practice, about the meaning of care. At every chance, I reworked academic assignments into publishable papers. Most appeared in *AJOT* as feature articles or persuasive pieces. Most drew from fictional and phenomenological literature, the arts, or history. Each humanities discipline helped my passion—the art of practice—grow.

When I later taught, I sought artistry in the classroom. I then wrote about confluent education, all the while infusing affective strands of learning into my students' work. Affective learning seemed a pathway to artful practice. Years later, I looked at research from its ethical and interpersonal sides, aspects of its artistry. I had no idea that these publications would lead me to the profession's ethos, the subject of my Eleanor Clarke Slagle Lecture. Nor did I know that my work would appear in physical therapy, physician assistant, and nursing literature venues that welcomed my voice.

My point in sharing is this: Finding voice can be a process. Only at some midway point could I name my developing voice. Finding voice was not a single event, a moment marked by a voice booming through parting clouds, *"This* shall be your fire." Bodies of work can grow from curiosity and learning. If you have an interest, you can raise a voice.

Nor is it ever too late to start writing. Surgeon and author Richard Selzer (2003) remembered, "Writing came to me late. I was 40 when I began to teach myself the arachnoid knack of spinning words" (p. 237). There is, of course, a strong likelihood of finding voice if a person is expert in some realm. Selzer's voice as a seasoned physician holds clout. Likewise, Slagle lecturers have voiced expertise, one affirmation of which is the published compendium of Slagle lectures *A Professional Legacy* (Padilla, 2005; Padilla & Griffiths, 2011). Most Slagle lecturers pulled from a body of work, a model of thought, a lifetime of practice. Examples across three decades make the point: Lilian Wegg (1960) wrote about work evaluation, Lela Llorens (1970) about human development, Alice Jantzen (1973) about occupational therapy education, and Robert K. Bing (1981) about occupational therapy history.

But the expertise of these therapists did not remove either the challenge or the work of writing. Each lecturer had to consider anew the matter of voice and how to honor the lectureship. In a foreword to the collection, I shared this view:

> The call to meet a need and push the profession forward in such a public way is at once a challenge and a privilege. . . . The privilege of the call draws one into deliberation about the best and the worst of the times. It invites one to find what one *can* say so as to make a difference. The import of the work fills each step along the way. Humility gives one frequent pause. (Peloquin, 2005b, p. xiii)

It can thus be said that giving voice even after it has been found is still work. It is the work of sharing ideas well, and that work occurs through the agency of style.

Giving Voice: The Importance of Writing Style

When a writer claims to be finding a voice at last, that statement includes not just discovery of a topic worth sharing but discovery of a writing style that works. It is writing style, that crafted "line of words," in Dillard's terms, which carries a writer's voice. A judicious or fortuitous union of idea and style shape for a writer a sense of "place" in writing. Just as a line of words can assume different forms to become miner's pick, carver's gouge, or surgeon's probe, diverse writing styles become a writer's tools.

Style in writing is commonly cast into three overarching types: narrative, expository, and persuasive. Seeking uniqueness of voice, writers learn to convey ideas using one or more of these styles. Dillard might call them narrative, expository, or persuasive "lines of words." Each writer writes distinctly, using fundamental styles. If spoken words carry personal traits such as precision, charm, or good timing, so does written text. If audible laughter ranges from guffaws to titters, so can a writer's wit. If verbal explanations unfold in dull or brilliant ways, so can a writer's prose. Let's spend time with each writing style, pausing to note where in the occupational therapy literature one can find examples.

NARRATIVE STYLE

A writer using narrative style tells the story of a personal or clinical event in either actual or fictional terms. The writer *narrates* the topic. Stories from leaders in occupational therapy have appeared in *AJOT* in "A Firm Persuasion in Our Work." Most are reflexive. Nedra Gillette (2008) told the story of the mentors who touched her life. Mary Law (2007) described her life as a journey shaped by curiosity. Susan Coppola (2005) shared her need to see the

> When a writer claims to be finding a voice at last, that statement includes not just discovery of a topic worth sharing but discovery of a writing style that works.

whole of things. Betty Abreu (2006) described her identity as linked with her workplaces. I shared a sense of coherence in longstanding occupations (Peloquin, 2006). Betty Hasselkus (2004) used this style well:

> During that first year of practice, I received a referral to treat a woman who had sustained severe burns over much of her body. The very limited range of motion she had in her upper extremities spurred me on to one of my first experiences of being innovative in therapy. I created a special spoon with a very long handle made from splinting material—riveted to the spoon and bent to just the right angle so that she could independently feed herself. I still remember the look of surprise and delight on her face when she brought the first spoonful of chili up to her mouth. After a few more spoonfuls, she began calling out to people going by in the hall to come and see what she could do. (p. 476)

Mary Higgins Clark (2003), author of mystery novels, used narrative style to explain why she writes:

> A common question asked of writers is, "When did you decide to become a writer?" The answer, of course, is that we didn't decide anything. It was decided for us. I firmly believe that mythical godmothers make appearance at our cradles, and bestow their gifts. The godmother who might have blessed me with a singing voice did not show up; the goddess of dance was nowhere in sight; the chef to the angels was otherwise engaged. Only one made the journey to my cradle, and she whispered, "You will be a storyteller." (p. 35)

EXPOSITORY STYLE

Writers using expository style approach a topic in an educational or explanatory way. The writer *expounds* or *explains* the topic, aiming to either convey information or shed light on obscure points. Researchers explain study results in this style. An example of expository writing appears in Wendy Coster's (2009) mindful discussion of measurement:

> Words connote reality. When we have extracted a pattern from the array of stimuli we experience, we mark the pattern with a name—a word. Almost immediately the word takes on the power to influence our thoughts and feelings. . . . Words reduce ambiguity to enable us to live socially in a world of objects. I can show you the object I give the name to, and we can agree to use that name whenever we speak about that object. Cultures vary in the extent to which they differentiate within particular categories, but they all have ways of marking or pointing out with words the features that differentiate the categories that are meaningful within their culture. (p. 743)

Practitioners who explain their practices do so in expository style. Some of their exposés appear in practice magazines as educational work. Writing in *OT Practice,* Guy McCormack (2009) revealed the aim of neuroscience:

> In essence, neuroscience studies have shown that learning and memory are the result of experience-driven alterations of the synaptic structures of neurons. Occupational therapy practitioners set up the circumstances and situations that modify the environment and the degree of challenge for a skill set (the *just-right challenge*) that creates an *adaptive response* that originates at the cellular and molecular level. In the clinic we cannot see this change at the cellular level but we do see measurable changes in behavior, memory, attention, and motor control. (p. CE-2)

Textbooks in occupational therapy curricula exemplify expository style. In those texts, writers make clear those constructs and skills that students must know. A paragraph from Kathlyn Reed's (2001) text illustrates this style while setting her book's tone:

> The purpose of this handbook is to provide students, practitioners, and researchers with a ready source of information about disorders or conditions seen in occupational therapy practice, as documented in published literature. Each disorder or condition is summarized using the same outline and headings. This consistency will allow for quick review and for comparison between topics. (p. vii)

Books cast in expository style target learners—new or lifelong—who hope to deepen their understanding of any focal area of practice, education, or research.

PERSUASIVE STYLE

Persuasive style aims to convince a reader that a perspective or action is worth taking. The writer *persuades*. In occupational therapy, one finds examples of this style in *AJOT*'s "The Issue Is" or "Nationally Speaking" sections. The words of Elizabeth Yerxa (1967) are persuasive:

> The authentic occupational therapist is open to the client's ideas and feelings and real in responding to them. He does not give in to the temptation to insulate himself against feeling because if he does so he will lose the capacity to be there. "Being there" also means being able to separate his feelings for the client as a human being from projections of how he would feel if he had experienced the client's disability. For the authentic occupational therapist knows that the client is the only one who can discover his own particular meaning. (p. 172)

Some readers have found my style persuasive. I did aim to persuade when writing this passage on spirituality:

> To see occupation as the making of lives and worlds is a deeper—and more spiritual—perspective than to see it as doing or performing. The image of someone in the act of making is one in which human being (character, heart, spirit) flows into human doing. The difference between doing and making is one of substance rather than semantic. . . . Occupation, the core of our therapy, animates and extends the human spirit; we participate in that animation. Gazing past the details of practice while led by their design to the point beyond, we discern a deeper aim. The discovery is awesome. (Peloquin, 1997, p. 168)

Persuasive writing can engender hope, inspire, or motivate. Persuasive works can provoke readers to thought and action; they can evoke deep feeling. Those who persuade write in a spirit of advocacy.

CHOOSING A STYLE

Part of giving voice to a topic well is to answer three style-based questions: Is there a story that I might tell? Is there something I know or do that I might explain? Is there an idea or action about which I can get persuasive? Answers to these questions will direct writers to their intentions and to their use of styles. Journalist and author Marie Arana (2003) said, "There are books that mark genius and books that shift gears. There are writers who plumb hearts and those who find doors" (p. 64); she was noting, in other words, the outcomes of style choices. When passion or authority drives style choices, writers and their works can be seen as agents in the world rather than as mere commentators. Narrative style can plumb hearts. Expository style can mark genius. Persuasive style can open doors. Each style can shift gears. The process of crafting a unique voice from among the various styles takes time and thought; it demands commitment to writing.

Commitment to the Occupation of Writing

If one is to find and give voice, then the right topic, congruent style, and unique mode of expression must come together. But they don't do so magically. A writer may claim that magical things happen in writing, but behind the magic is commitment to the craft. I vividly recall one magical time while writing my Slagle lecture. I had been working on the two halves of the paper at once, attending to the history of our ethos—our guiding beliefs—as well as to the challenge of enacting such beliefs in modern times. I had honed my wording of the five guiding beliefs to these:

> **A writer may claim that magical things happen in writing, but behind the magic is commitment to the craft.**

1. "Time, place, and circumstance open paths to occupation."
2. "Occupation fosters dignity, competence, and health."
3. "Occupational therapy is a personal engagement."
4. "Caring and helping are vital to the work."
5. "Effective practice is artistry and science." (Peloquin, 2005a, p. 623)

As I tracked between the halves of the paper seeking a bridge, I was suddenly struck by an idea so fitting that I literally danced in place. For each belief statement, I could craft a matching affirmation! A series of affirmations about "who we are" might let practitioners hear our ethos as a calling. These affirmations have since appeared on T-shirts in many occupational therapy programs:

1. "We are pathfinders."
2. "We enable occupations that heal."
3. "We cocreate daily lives."
4. "We reach for hearts as well as hands."
5. "We are artists and scientists at once." (Peloquin, 2005a, p. 623)

I have "felt the magic" when I've been so deeply pressed—on all sides and from within—by ideas and words that a sudden burst of possibility, a brilliance of thought, a wave of high energy have lifted me to higher ground. The work—hours spent thinking, wordsmithing, foraging for images, and dabbling in rich ideas—incubates the magic.

In a palm-sized book entitled *Children's Letters to God* (Hample & Marshall, 1991), young Lois shared her angst about writing: "Dear God, I like the Lord's prayer best of all. Did you have to write it a lot, or did you get it right the first time? I have to write everything I ever write over again." The effort of writing well is clear to anyone who has tried. Dillard (1989), remember, likened writing to digging underground, carving wood, and cutting into bodies. Her take on the effort is clear: "Out of a human population on earth of four billion, perhaps twenty people can write a serious book in a year. Some people lift cars, too" (p. 13). Because lifting cars seems so daunting, I'll propose three doable acts to which an aspiring writer can commit: reading good writing, rewriting, and using precise words.

COMMIT TO READING GOOD WRITING

If you want to write well, commit to reading good writing. When students study samples of good documentation, they write better notes. Likewise, good writing teaches sentence structure and syntax. Good writing teaches rhythm and pace. Good writing enlarges vocabulary. When a reader attends to a well-written piece, many lessons follow. Writer and political activist Nadine Gordimer (2003) said, "The only school for a writer is the library—reading, reading. . . . Learning from other writers' perceptions that you have to find your way to yours, at the urge of the most powerful sense of yourself—creativity. Apart from that, you're on your own" (p. 60).

I am struck by the lessons found in pithy chapter titles in some books on writing. In listing a few here, I hope to pique curiosity and prompt reflection; both can fuel commitment. First, from *The Writing Life* (Arana, 2003), consider these:

- "The Seduction of the Text," by Francine Du Plessix Gray
- "Doing It for Love," by Erica Jong
- "The Writer as Outlaw," by Jayne Anne Phillips
- "Sounds and Sensibilities," by Ned Rorem
- "Writer, Be Afraid," by Michael Chabon.

Each is provocative, is it not? And each chapter is equally instructive. Occupational therapists can read about writing just as they read about splinting or low-fat cooking. And what fun to learn more about seductive texts or outlaw practices!

These next chapter titles, from *Writers on Writing: Collected Essays From the New York Times* (Darnton, 2001), are in themselves whimsical lessons:

- "To Engage the World More Fully, Follow a Dog," by Rick Bass
- "From Echoes Emerge Original Voices," by Nicholas Delbanco
- "The Enduring Commitment of a Faithful Storyteller," by Maureen Howard
- "Comforting Lessons in Arranging Life's Details," by David Leavitt
- "Directions: Write, Read, Rewrite. Repeat Steps 2 and 3 as Needed," by Susan Sontag.

Much is written to help those who would write. Susan Sontag (2001) said, "Reading usually precedes writing. And the impulse to write is almost always fired by reading. Reading, the love of reading, is what makes you dream of becoming a writer" (p. 226). Long ago, writer and editor Dorothea Brande (1934) offered a suggestion that still works for me:

> Read with every faculty alert. Notice the rhythm of the book, and whether it accelerated or slowed down when the author wished to be emphatic. Look for mannerisms or favorite words, and decide for yourself whether they are worth trying for practice or whether they are too plainly the author's own to reward you for learning their structure. (p. 103)

COMMIT TO REWRITING

If you want to write well, commit to rewriting. It surprises me when a student submits a draft as a finished paper. My 10th drafts are still works in progress. Over the years, my rewriting has become a clear enough process for me to call it *sculpting*. At first, long sentences bear my unraveling thoughts. I revise the text to shorten it, trying to get the rhythm right. If I sense the need for one syllable and not three, my choice of *motivate* might change to *press*. I scan paragraphs for rhythm, too, so that short sentences stand near longer ones. Brevity lends power. It also gives pause. Dillard's carving metaphor fits the sculpting that I do. With each rewrite, more falls away, and my message gets clear. I see the work as "starting to sing" when ideas and words are meshing well. There's excitement at this stage. Susan Sontag (2001) felt the joy: "And though this, the rewriting—and the rereading—sound like effort, they are actually the most pleasurable parts of writing" (p. 224).

I did not always sculpt my text. I first felt the rhythm in words as I wrote my dissertation, when I also sought their precise use. A passage from my first published article in 1988 on the incorporation into occupational therapy of a psychological construct called *therapy set*, now seems awkward:

> Although the purpose of this article is not to investigate the effectiveness of enlightening patients about and involving them in their therapy, but to explore a rationale for the use of such a collaborative approach in occupational therapy, some brief discussion of the effectiveness of the approach seems indicated. (Peloquin, 1988, p. 775)

I would write the same thoughts differently now, perhaps like this:

> My aim is to propose therapy set as a means of helping patients collaborate. Research in psychology has shown that therapy set gives patients vital information that leads to their engagement. These studies make a good starting point.

COMMIT TO USING PRECISE WORDS

If you want to write well, commit to using precise words. The phrase *le mot juste* in French roughly translates as "the just-right word." Words that convey a writer's meaning precisely are key to finding and giving voice. Only the right word carries the topic truly. Only the right word conveys intent clearly. Precise words seem a matter of integrity. I often sit with students who tell me what they meant to say because their writing did not. When I ask them to read aloud what they have written, *aha!*s and recanting often follow. I suggest that they write until they capture what they mean to say. What one says precisely is often said uniquely. Again I borrow wisdom from Dorothea Brande (1934):

> It is well to understand in one's writing life that there is just one contribution which every one of us can make: we can give into the common pool of experience some comprehension of the world as it looks to each of us. There is one sense in which everyone is unique. No one else was born of your parents, at just that time of just that country's history; no one underwent just your experiences, reached just your conclusions, or faces the world with the exact set of ideas that you must have. If you . . . are willing to say precisely what you think of any situation . . . you will inevitably have a piece of work that is original. (p. 121)

Barbara DeMarco-Barrett (2004) said that she harvests words, arguing that only if one has many words at hand can one say what one means. A large vocabulary, one that DeMarco-Barrett would call "splendid," solidifies a writer's line of words. She described writers who collect words in notebooks as they read. I keep dictionaries near my phone, making discoveries while the phone rings or I'm on hold. DeMarco-Barrett found five new words a day:

> I love words. Most writers love words. The feel of them on the tongue. Round sounds, sharp sounds, clicking sounds. . . . When a writer has given new life to words you've heard a million times before or uses words you don't use or ordinarily think of but love, it's inspiring. (p. 31)

This discussion of commitment to using precise words now comes full circle: back to reading. The best way to learn about words, to see how they work in precise and awesome ways, comes back to the first commitment that I proposed. You may not have to lift cars, but you really *must* read!

Venues and Affirmations: Contexts That Carry Voice Forward

It would be nice to think that a writer who writes well and with passion will find both venue and affirmation. That outcome appears not always to be the case. Annie Dillard (1989) said it well: "This writing that you do, that so thrills you, that so rocks and exhilarates you, as if you were dancing next to the band, is barely audible to anyone else" (p. 17). But venues and readers soon matter to a writer, one way or another. Even if the act of writing is meaningful, without readers, a voice goes unheard. Erica Jong (2003) said, "Writers are born to voice what we all feel. That is the gift. And we keep it alive by giving it away" (p. 67). In the absence of some venue, a voice can't be heard, and there will be no gift.

First writing attempts are said to teach much to many about venue and validation. My first attempt was instructive. When I submitted my first piece, on therapy set, to *AJOT* (Peloquin, 1988), one review was positive. But because the other proposed rejection, I dropped all thoughts of seeing that paper in print. Months later, then-editor Elaine Viseltear called, asking about my plans to resubmit. I was stunned. When I told her that one reviewer had made that plan seem foolhardy, she said that I wrote well, that the journal needed mental health articles, and that I had a sound message. Had I not gotten that call, I'm not sure I'd have written again. As it turned out, I have published 33 articles in *AJOT,* a venue in which most readers have found my work.

From this experience I learned that reviewers can be helpful mentors who support emerging writers. Any review connotes a second look; it aims to view the work anew. A good reviewer holds the writer in high regard. Standing outside the written work, good reviewers give perspective, share knowledge, and offer counsel. They shepherd apt revisions when those may be helpful or open doors to better venues when that action seems best. Reviewers who slip away from mentoring to act as gatekeepers can squelch early efforts. Mindful of the publisher, they nearly snub the writer. When such a slip occurs, opportunity is lost. At its best, the review process is a sharing of keen perspectives. At its worst, it is a withholding of hope.

Writers must be open to critical feedback without being crushed by its impact. I love the way in which Mary Higgins Clark (2003) put feedback and affirmation in perspective:

> Letters from readers can be gratifying and heartwarming. But I think my all-time favorite came from a 13–year-old who wrote:
>
> > Dear Mrs. Clark:
> > I have read the first half of *Where Are the Children*.
> > You are a wonderful writer.
> > Someday I hope to read the second half.
> > Your friend, Jack. (p. 38)

Erica Jong (2003) shared this helpful view: "I was blessed to encounter criticism early. It forced me to listen to my inner voice, not to the roar of the crowd. This is the most useful lesson a writer can learn" (p. 68). It's perhaps best to get philosophical about feedback and to think of it as hearing back from select readers. It's a given that not all readers will want to read what you write, let alone benefit from it. Accepting that fact seems wise.

Time spent writing is time spent trying. Novelist George Pelecanos (2003) said,

> When I speak to groups of students in public schools, I tell them that, 25 years ago, I was exactly where they are today. I want to demystify all this, make them see that whatever they want in life is within their grasp. But they have to take the first steps. They have to try. (p. 88)

Annie Dillard (1989) agreed:

> Rembrandt and Shakespeare, Tolstoy and Gauguin, possessed, I believe, powerful hearts, not powerful wills. They loved the range of materials they used. . . . They worked, respectfully, out of their love and knowledge, and they produced complex bodies of work that endure. Then and only then, the world flapped at them some sort of hat, which, if they were still living, they ignored as well as they could, to keep at their tasks. (p. 71)

Here's my counsel if you hope to publish: Study publications for the article types they hold. Engage editors in conversation about the fit of a work you're writing. Call editors for a better perspective on reviews that seem harsh. Consider special issues and special sections as fine places to start. Learn from others about different venues. And remember that some venues are simply better places for your work than others. Finding these early can save you time.

Another source of affirmation for a writer is cowriting. Writing with others is a good and gentle source of feedback. Any combination of teamwork is possible, because cowriting invites a sharing of gifts and distribution of work. One writer may have the right style and the other the deep passion. Both may share a passion equally, with one more inclined to write. One may be seasoned and the other hoping to learn. Even solo writers can benefit from the affirmation that comes from collaboration; I have done so on several occasions. Cowriting can yield a harmony of voices not possible in solo work.

Finding Voice, Accepting Grace

My last comments about voice take me to the matter of grace. As I noted earlier, there are moments when the writing process takes over, as if one has truly become occupied by—lived in by—the words and ideas that one writes. Given over to such engagement, a writer receives much. I felt my experience as a near-magical burst of possibility, brilliance, and energy. Dillard (1989) described the gift well:

> At its best, the sensation of writing is that of any unmerited grace. It is handed to you, but only if you look for it. You search, you break your heart, your back, your brain, and then—and only then—it is handed to you. (p. 75)

When such grace is given, the urge is to pass it on—to give it away. For this reason, I've entitled this chapter "Finding Your Voice and Giving It Away."

The strongest affirmation that you will get in writing comes from the belief that you have labored well and that your work can be a gift. That belief resonates well with Whyte's (2001) words. Hear them again: "to feel that what we do is right for ourselves and good for the world at the same time—is one of the great triumphs of human existence" (p. 4). If you have been flirting with the idea of writing, my hope is that the lines of words in this chapter will nudge you closer to this point of persuasion: You really must try!

> **The strongest affirmation that you will get in writing comes from the belief that you have labored well and that your work can be a gift.**

REFERENCES

Abreu, B. C. (2006). A Firm Persuasion in Our Work—Professional identity and workplace integration. *American Journal of Occupational Therapy, 60,* 596–599.

Alvarez, J. (2003). On finding a Latino voice. In M. Arana (Ed.), *The writing life: Writers on how they think and work* (pp. 128–133). New York: Public Affairs.

Arana, M. (Ed.). (2003). *The writing life: Writers on how they think and work.* New York: Public Affairs.

Ayres, A. J. (1963). The development of perceptual–motor abilities: A theoretical basis for treatment of dysfunction. *American Journal of Occupational Therapy, 17,* 221–225.

Bing, R. K. (1981). Occupational therapy revisited: A paraphrastic journey (Eleanor Clarke Slagle Lecture). *American Journal of Occupational Therapy, 35,* 499–518.

Brande, D. (1934). *Becoming a writer.* New York: Harcourt, Brace & Company.

Clark, M. H. (2003). Touched by an angel. In M. Arana (Ed.), *The writing life: Writers on how they think and work* (pp. 35–38). New York: Public Affairs.

Coppola, S. (2005). A Firm Persuasion in Our Work—A journey to see the whole of things. *American Journal of Occupational Therapy, 59,* 476–479.

Cornwell, P. (2003). The passionate researcher. In M. Arana (Ed.), *The writing life: Writers on how they think and work* (pp. 152–155). New York: Public Affairs.

Coster, W. J. (2009). Embracing ambiguity: Facing the challenge of measurement (Eleanor Clarke Slagle Lecture). *American Journal of Occupational Therapy, 62,* 743–752.

Darnton, J. (2001). *Writers on writing: Collected essays from the New York Times.* New York: Times Books.

DeMarco-Barrett, B. (2004). *Pen on fire: A busy woman's guide to igniting the writer within.* Orlando, FL: Harcourt.

Dillard, A. (1989). *The writing life.* New York: Harper & Row.

Gillette, N. (2008). A Firm Persuasion in Our Work—Mentors I have known (and loved). *American Journal of Occupational Therapy, 61,* 487–490.

Gordimer, N. (2003). Being a product of your dwelling place. In M. Arana (Ed.), *The writing life: Writers on how they think and work* (pp. 59–63). New York: Public Affairs.

Hample, S., & Marshall, E. (1991). *Children's letters to God.* New York: Workman.

Hasselkus, B. R. (2004). A Firm Persuasion in Our Work—Deeper into the heart of the matter. *American Journal of Occupational Therapy, 58,* 476–479.

Iwama, M. K. (2005). The Kawa (river) model: Nature, life flow, and the power of culturally relevant occupational therapy. In F. Kronenberg, S. Algado, & N. Pollard (Eds.), *Occupational therapy without borders: Learning from the spirit of survivors* (pp. 213–227). London: Elsevier/Churchill Livingstone.

Jantzen, A. C. (1973). Academic occupational therapy: A career specialty (Eleanor Clarke Slagle Lecture). *American Journal of Occupational Therapy, 27,* 1–7.

Jong, E. (2003). Doing it for love. In M. Arana (Ed.), *The writing life: Writers on how they think and work* (pp. 66–70). New York: Public Affairs.

Law, M. C. (2007). A Firm Persuasion in Our Work—Occupational therapy: A journey driven by curiosity. *American Journal of Occupational Therapy, 61,* 599–602.

Llorens, L. A. (1970). Facilitating growth and development: The promise of occupational therapy (Eleanor Clarke Slagle Lecture). *American Journal of Occupational Therapy, 24,* 93–101.

McCormack, G. L. (2009, September 28). How occupational therapy influences neuroplasticity. *OT Practice, 14*(17), CE-1–CE-8.

Padilla, R. (Ed.). (2005). *A professional legacy: The Eleanor Clarke Slagle Lectures in occupational therapy, 1955–2004.* Bethesda, MD: AOTA Press.

Padilla, R., & Griffiths, Y. (Eds.). (2011). *A professional legacy: The Eleanor Clarke Slagle Lectures in occupational therapy, 1995–2010.* Bethesda, MD: AOTA Press.

Pelecanos, G. P. (2003). Between origins and art. In M. Arana (Ed.), *The writing life: Writers on how they think and work* (pp. 85–89). New York: Public Affairs.

Peloquin, S. M. (1988). Linking purpose to procedure during interactions with patients. *American Journal of Occupational Therapy, 42,* 775–781.

Peloquin, S. M. (1997). The spiritual depth of occupation: Making worlds and making lives. *American Journal of Occupational Therapy, 51,* 167–168.

Peloquin, S. M. (2005a). Embracing our ethos, reclaiming our heart (Eleanor Clarke Slagle Lecture). *American Journal of Occupational Therapy, 59,* 611–625.

Peloquin, S. M. (2005b). Foreword. In R. Padilla (Ed.), *A professional legacy: The Eleanor Clarke Slagle Lectures in occupational therapy* (p. xiii). Bethesda, MD: AOTA Press.

Peloquin, S. M. (2006). A Firm Persuasion in Our Work—Occupations: Strands of coherence in a life. *American Journal of Occupational Therapy, 60,* 236–239.

Reed, K. L. (2001). *Quick reference to occupational therapy.* Austin, TX: Pro-Ed.

Selzer, R. (2003). Writer with scalpel. In M. Arana (Ed.), *The writing life: Writers on how they think and work* (pp. 237–241). New York: Public Affairs.

Sontag, S. (2001). Directions: Write, read, rewrite. Repeat steps 2 and 3 as needed. In J. Darnton (Ed.), *Writers on writing: Collected essays from the New York Times* (pp. 223–229). New York: Henry Holt.

Townsend, E., & Whiteford, G. (2005). A participatory occupational justice framework: Population-based processes of practice. In F. Kronenberg, S. Algado, & N. Pollard (Eds.), *Occupational therapy without borders: Learning from the spirit of survivors* (pp. 110–126). London: Elsevier/Churchill Livingstone.

Wegg, L. S. (1960). The essentials of work evaluation (Eleanor Clarke Slagle Lecture). *American Journal of Occupational Therapy, 14,* 65–69, 79.

Whyte, D. (2001). *Crossing the unknown sea: Work as a pilgrimage of identity.* New York: Riverhead.

Wood, W. (2005). A Firm Persuasion in Our Work—Associate editor's note. *American Journal of Occupational Therapy, 59,* 107.

Yerxa, E. J. (1967). Authentic occupational therapy (Eleanor Clarke Slagle Lecture). *American Journal of Occupational Therapy, 21,* 155–173.

Getting Started

4

Refreshing, Renewing, and Remediating Your Writing: Back to the Basics

RONDALYN V. WHITNEY, PhD, OT/L

We are as much informed of a writer's genius by what he selects as by what he originates.

—RALPH WALDO EMERSON (N.D.)

Writing is the process of discovering ideas, making connections, creating new perspectives, demanding something new from a reader, creating a new world through transcribed ideas, and empowering thought through the written word. Writing is simultaneously a powerful process and an innovative act. Throughout history, writers have evoked passionate change, agitated for revolutionary ideas, and often been the first to be eliminated when new powers take over. Words can make you laugh, weep, or open your wallet and contribute to a cause; they can take you to

> Words can make you laugh, weep, or open your wallet and contribute to a cause; they can take you to imagined worlds, make you see history in a new light, and change paradigms.

imagined worlds, make you see history in a new light, and change paradigms.

All good writing, whether politically activating or documenting a procedure for reimbursement, relies on the writer's skill. Skill develops over time and wanes with disuse. Knitters may already know how to cast on but not how to purl, or they may want to refresh their memory of the basic stitches after a long hiatus from weaving yarns into scarves, socks, or baby blankets. Similarly, although most adults know how to write, an aspiring writer needs to update and expand his or her basic knowledge to write well.

The technical basics of writing form the foundation on which creative, coherent pieces of written work rest. Writers need to update the tools in their toolkit, follow a process for using those tools to communicate effectively, and improve their skills over time.

Tools in Your Writing Toolkit

Artists, crafters, and hobbyists use tools. A knitter needs yarn, needles, and a gauge. A chef needs sharp knives, a perfectly seasoned sauté pan, and fresh herbs or infused oils. A writer needs words, sentences, paragraphs, and sections.

WORDS

The most important tool for a writer is vocabulary. I once had a student who was convinced I could read his mind because I could tell when he had used the synonym feature of Microsoft Word. How? He had selected the wrong choice for the intent of the text. *Word choice* is how an artist wields the tool of vocabulary. Mary Reilly (1962) could have said, "Using their hands keeps people healthy"; instead, she said, "Man, through the use of his hands, as they are energized by mind and will, can influence the state of his own health" (p. 1). Reilly's version, although less concise, is richer in clarity of detail.

Building a Rich Vocabulary

Building a vocabulary can feel like a task, a chore you had hoped to be rid of after passing your college entrance exams. But a rich vocabulary eases the writing process, and playing with vocabulary allows you to have fun while amassing an arsenal of just-right words. Challenge yourself with crosswords, Will Shortz (1996, 2004) puzzles, and other word-related games. As you write, a good thesaurus will help you a great deal, but a dictionary is still a writer's best friend. A dictionary provides usage information, an explanation of how synonyms differ in use, and ideally, the etymology of a word.

Keep a small notebook, and write down words (or add them to a notes app or feature of your phone) that have piqued your interest. Later, you can look them up, record their definition, and endeavor to use them whenever possible. Words like *avuncular, prodigious,* and *paradoxical* were such words for me years ago. I call these *million-dollar words,* words that, if appropriate to your audience, are more specific and expressive than their more common counterparts *nice, amazing,* and *confusing.* Also collect words that you think sound musical or that produce a pleasant feeling when you say them, like *quixotic, undulating,* or *tantalizing.*

Using such words in your writing helps you talk about your pursuits in a way that sounds just as passionate as you are. Review your list weekly; if you learn one word a week, you'll amass 52 words a year—not a bad collection!

Another category of million-dollar words are those that involve the senses. Occupational therapy practitioners are trained to value the contributions of the sensory system to participation in the occupations of everyday life. Sensory terms provide readers with a visceral understanding of your message. For example, if you want to describe a landscape, you can say it is green (sight), loud (hearing), fragrant (smell), sweet (taste), and lush (feeling), as in "The mountains of Appalachia are green, loudly towering in the distance, and the trees fragrant, sweet, and lush." You can use your million-dollar words and say, "The mountains of Appalachia are emeralds, resounding in the distance, the pungent smell of ancient loam luxuriantly permeating the air." If you really want to milk the senses, include vestibular and proprioceptive detail and add, "I am rendered dizzy by the heaviness of nature's majestic blanket." Now to apply it to a client, who smiled (sight) and laughed (sound) with peers but withdrew and began to hum to herself when the chilled (touch) grape (smell) play dough was offered to the group. Or, a client can have flushed cheeks (sight), recoil from texture (touch), scream that a teacher stinks (smell) when she smells like eucalyptus,

Sensory terms provide readers with a visceral understanding of your message.

cover his ears in music class when recorders are played (sound), lick nonfood items (taste), or move with an awkward gait (movement).

In one section of the word list, at the top of each page write *Tactile, Olfactory, Gustatory, Auditory, Visual,* and *Movement/Weight* (for vestibular and proprioceptive). As you come across words that fit these categories, add them to your collection. Two excellent books about sensory writing are writer and poet Diane Ackerman's (1990) book *A Natural History of the Senses* and occupational therapist Winnie Dunn's (2008) *Living Sensationally: Understanding Your Senses.* Figure 4.1 provides a brief exercise to help you practice using sensory words.

Using Pronouns Appropriately

A final way to enrich your word choice is to avoid overrelying on pronouns. Pronouns have their place—they enable you to avoid repeating the noun—but you should use them sparingly, and only when the reader can clearly understand what they refer to. Carol Kranowitz, a preschool teacher and prolific author on sensory-processing disorder, edited my first book and caught me overusing the word *it.* I have worked to use *it* as little as possible in my writing, forcing me to take the time to be specific in what I say.

Pronouns must agree in person (e.g., second person [you] vs. third person [he or she]) and in number (singular vs. plural) with the noun they refer to; for example, if one sentence refers to "students," the next one should speak about "they," not "you." Pronouns can be a challenge to master, especially for nonnative English speakers. Two key rules are important to remember: (1) Make sure you keep an eye on agreement on first, second, and third person throughout your paragraphs to avoid confusing your reader, and (2) craft your sentences to avoid pronouns (and nouns) that appear sexist. For example, if Mary Reilly's sentence quoted earlier in this chapter were published today, *a person* would probably be substituted for *man* and *his or her* for *his* to avoid the appearance of bias.

SENTENCES

Sentences have a structure. They all need an actor (subject) and an action (verb): *Trees grow. The patient dressed.* Descriptors, selected with care from your ever-growing vocabulary, make the sentence more vivid and precise: *California trees grow tall. The patient dressed slowly.* The rules for turning your words into sentences are called *grammar* and *mechanics,* and a writer

The purpose of this exercise is to show that by thinking about the sensory aspects of even the most mundane object, a richness evolves in writing. Try thinking about the senses as you write; you might be surprised what emerges from your pen.

Find an object in your environment, like a coffee mug, your cat, or your toes. Now, fill in the blanks.

Think of the five senses and of movement:

It looks like _____.
It feels like _____.
It smells like _____.
It sounds like _____.
It tastes like _____.
It moves like _____.

Connect the object with what you know:

It reminds me of _____ because it _____.

Observe and record causes and effects:

When I _____, it _____.

Note any changes:

It changed after _____, and now it _____.

Be curious:

I am curious about _____.
I wonder what would happen if _____.

Here's an example:

Earl Grey tea at night

It looks like milk candy.
It feels like autumn.
It smells like winter blossoms.
It sounds like stillness after a storm.
It tastes like nightfall.
It moves like a vortex, gravity pulling down to the bottom of the mug, to times past.
It reminds me of Sunday mornings in New England, because I discovered the warmth of long brunches with new friends, over pots and pots of tea.
When I take a sip, I am reminded that nothing matters but this moment, infinite.
It changed after I moved inland, and now I have tea as I sit cozy in my favorite chair each evening, my transition to relaxation after long days.
I am curious about bergamot—how something so exotic became my daily brew.
I wonder what would happen if I held the warm mug close to my ear. Would I hear the sounds of the ocean, two decades ago, watching storms off the coast of Marblehead?

FIGURE 4.1. Using sensory words.

New writers seem to think "good" writers do not need to consult references, but that is far from the truth. Experienced writers have shelves full of reference guides. Don't hesitate to do some investigating for your own growth as a writer.

has to follow those rules or suffer the consequences: Readers either won't understand you or may find it too cumbersome to discern the meaning in your words (or both). And you can count on this: Instructors will give you a lower grade, and editors will reject your manuscripts if you have a lot of grammatical or mechanical errors!

Learning Grammar

Grammar refers to rules about tense, word order, and subject–verb agreement. Grammar can be complex to learn completely, but it is easy to (re)learn enough of the basics to be a good writer. In my experience, grammatical and mechanical errors are signs that your thoughts got ahead of your writing. If you want to brush up on grammar and mechanics, buy or borrow a good book on grammar, or find a good Web site. I recommend *Woe Is I: The Grammarphobe's Guide to Better English in Plain English* by professional editor Patricia O'Connor (1998) as a fun way to review grammar.

For a more in-depth refresher, learn how to diagram sentences (this once-required elementary school ritual has given way to the modern "language arts"). This system of literally drawing out the elements of a sentence teaches you to see language as it pieces together into well-crafted, grammatically sound sentences. Communications maven Nan DeVincent-Hayes's (1995) workbook *Grammar and Diagramming Sentences* reviews sentence structure and provides practice in diagramming. If you prefer online learning, hundreds of Web sites will guide you through the process.

Understanding the Mechanics

Mechanics refers to established conventions in spelling, capitalization, and punctuation. Like the rules of grammar, the rules of mechanics have to be learned, practiced, and relearned. You may want to acquire two or three good references and consult them when you have a question. New writers seem to think "good" writers do not need to consult references, but that is far from the truth. Experienced writers have shelves full of reference guides. Don't hesitate to do some investigating for your own growth as a writer. Consult the dictionary with questions on spelling (your spell-checker is usually, but not always, reliable). One style guide you probably use often (e.g., American Psychological Association, 2010; Gibaldi, 2008) provides summaries of capitalization and punctuation rules. A fun read on mechanics in general is *Eats, Shoots and Leaves: The Zero Tolerance Approach to Punctuation* by writer Lynn Truss (2004). Be mindful, however, that as you learn the rules of mechanics and grammar, and become more sensitive to errors, you will hear a lot of people who *should* know better making mistakes!

PARAGRAPHS

A *paragraph* is a group of sentences that discuss a single idea or point. Each paragraph should begin with a topic sentence that introduces an idea that supports your thesis or the point you are trying to make with your writing. The middle sentences provide that support by giving examples and analyzing the significance of these examples. The last sentence of the paragraph can be used to draw a conclusion for that supporting idea or to transition to the next paragraph.

After you finish writing your paper, reread it and check each paragraph to see if there is more than one idea or point in that paragraph. If you find this, break that paragraph into two or three, one each for the points you find. If two paragraphs discuss exactly the same idea or point, combine them into one and trim unnecessary verbiage, or tweak them so they discuss two different aspects of the same idea or point.

SECTIONS

All writing needs a structure if you want to present your ideas in a logical order, otherwise the discussion winds around and away from the concepts, creating a dizzying, entangled swirl for the reader. The structure (and the length of its components) can vary, depending on the purpose of and audience for the paper. You can adapt the following three-section generic structure to your specific writing project: (1) an introduction that includes a thesis statement (your main idea), (2) body paragraphs that provide supporting details, and (3) a conclusion that restates the take-away points for readers.

The *introduction* gives background information on your topic, explains why your audience should be interested, and lays the groundwork for your thesis statement. Think of the introduction as your *hook:* you want to grab your reader's attention. The *thesis statement,* usually confined to one sentence, orients the reader to the main idea you will address in the paper. It doesn't matter if you write the introduction before or after you write the body of your essay; writers have different preferences. You can draft the introduction first and then revise and focus it once you have written the body or start with a well-developed introduction and move on from there. However, you should *always* start with a thesis statement, even a draft, so the rest of your writing is organized around the salient ideas.

The *body* of the paper consists of a series of paragraphs, each with a separate topic sentence and supporting ideas, and the paragraphs should work together to support and follow your thesis statement. Remember, each paragraph will follow the rule of threes (topic, support, conclusion). If you are writing a longer paper, you may wish to divide the body into subsections with headings to orient the reader. Think of the each heading as a topic that must relate to your thesis statement.

The *conclusion* often is the most difficult section to write. Many writers think that they have nothing left to say after having written the paper. Keep in mind that the conclusion is often what a reader remembers best; consider ending with a question or a provocative statement. Give the reader something to think about, perhaps a way to use your paper in the real world. If your introduction went from general to specific, steer your conclusion from specific to general. A common error is to simply repeat what was your paper. Instead take the opportunity to stress the importance of the thesis statement, giving the paper a sense of completeness and leaving a final impression with the reader.

The Writing Process

English professors Peter Elbow (2008) and Diana Hacker (2006), as well as the National Writing Project (www.nwp.org), and many others, have described the writing process in different ways, but they all agree that writing needs to be planned, shaped, and given time for polishing through revision and editing. This section discusses a five-part process useful for a wide variety of writing projects: (1) shape your idea, make a plan; (2) develop your thesis statement; (3) write the first draft; (4) revise; and (5) proofread.

1. SHAPE YOUR IDEA, MAKE A PLAN

Before you begin to put words to the page, take the time to plan a structure for your paper. A structure helps you organize your thoughts and write efficiently. It also helps you avoid frustration, paralysis, and procrastination (see Chapter 8, this volume, on overcoming procrastination).

When you develop your outline, organize your main points and supporting ideas and decide the best order with which to present them to the reader. Developing an outline is hard work, and many are tempted to skip this step, to the detriment of their project. If you're having trouble creating an outline, try one of the techniques writers use to get ideas going, often referred to as *prewriting techniques.* For example, *mind mapping* suggests you jot down your ideas (summarized in a few words) on a piece of blank paper as they occur to you, drawing lines between them to show how they are linked. You end up with a graphic representation of your ideas that can be turned into an outline.

Free writing involves writing whatever comes to mind, without worrying about grammar or mechanics; what you write may be unusable, but it gets your thinking going and enables you to move forward with your outline. Other techniques include *brainstorming*—talking through your idea aloud, discussing your idea with friends, and doing whatever gives you inspiration (e.g., taking a walk, reading your favorite author, listening to music). You want to decide how to organize your material—you can organize your thoughts around an image, like spinning a web, or around a calendar, taking the reader through the birth of an idea (spring), blossoming (summer), harvest (fall), and quiet reflection (winter).

Having a structure helps you to organize your thoughts. Honing your craft requires taking several steps. Like refinishing a table—sanding off the old finish, wiping off the dust, applying the new color, and letting the stain dry before applying lacquer—writing follows a process, an order, and a structure. When you're frustrated and don't know what step to take next, you can become paralyzed—unable to move forward—and procrastinate.

2. DEVELOP YOUR THESIS STATEMENT

The *thesis statement* is a one-sentence summary of the main idea or centralizing point of your paper and appears at or near the end of the introduction. Your thesis statement announces your intention—makes a promise, if you will, to the reader—and suggests the emphasis, direction, and scope of the paper that will follow. If well crafted, your thesis statement will capture the interest of the audience and whet their curiosity about the topic at hand.

The thesis statement typically is a work in progress, refined with each revision to make a fresher, more interesting, and more original advanced organizer for the rest of the written piece. I find it helpful to think of the key points you will make in your writing; include those in your thesis statement, and use those points to unify your essay.

3. WRITE THE FIRST DRAFT

After the first two steps, you have an outline and a draft thesis statement. Now, and only now, are you ready to write. Give yourself enough time to let your thoughts simmer and bubble to the top of your mind. Find a comfortable place to do your writing—a space free of the distractions that remind you of the million other things you could be doing. For example, noise doesn't distract me, but I can't tolerate clutter. My husband, however, wears earplugs when he has to create something, but he can ignore piles of toys and laundry and a week's worth of dishes.

There are at least two methods for writing your ideas down: author Kurt Vonnegut (1998) called those who use them *swoopers* and *bashers*. Swoopers prefer to get all their thoughts out quickly in a gush, a regurgitation; they splatter ideas across the page with little attention to grammar, mechanics, or style. Later, they return and craft the language, color-coding passages, excising lines, and cutting their own work without self-pity. Bashers, in contrast, painstakingly fix every word, every line, each idea before they move on to the next. When they are finished, they are done, having hammered every piece into place. As you can imagine, bashers are harder to edit because they argue for each hard-earned word. Swoopers are hard to edit because they can overwhelm you in the aftermath of their prose bombs.

I have substituted Vonnegut's term *swooper* with *slasher*. I think it better describes one who paints with a broad stroke and then slashes away the excess. Slashers and bashers work well together to produce written documents if the basher refrains from judging the slasher's meandering ways and the slasher proceeds gently with recommendations to alter the bashed-and-hashed precision of the basher's text.

No matter what kind of process you use to get your thoughts down on paper, when you write, consider your audience, and pay attention to the appropriateness of your tone. *Tone* conveys the attitude of a paper. For example, serious, frivolous, intimate, formal, informal, detached, or objective are each unique *tones*. The objective tone is most appropriate for academic and professional writing. Match your tone to your audience, always, even in an e-mail. A professor merits a formal tone, as does a potential future employer or an editor. An overly informal cover letter will take you out of consideration for a job, for example, whereas an overly formal note to a friend will cause him or her to wonder if you really are a friend. I had a boyfriend once who signed his valentine card to me "Best, Max Dickson." We had been dating 2 years, and the formal tone of his words struck me as odd (and turned out to be an omen).

4. REVISE

Now that you have your thoughts down on paper, it's time to take another look at what you have written and make changes to enhance the logic of the structure; clarify the ideas and make sure that they flow well from one to another. You can work to improve the introduction, thesis statement, and conclusion, and delete anything that doesn't fit. Exceptional papers have been revised at least twice; use the final revision to assure no further changes to the content are necessary and to correct any errors in grammar and mechanics.

5. PROOFREAD

Proofreading is the final step. You or someone who really cares about you (or owes you) can read to check for typographical errors. One good way to proof your own paper without getting lost in the content is to slowly read your work aloud or even backward; in these instances, typos will jump out at you more easily. If possible, exchange papers with a friend to proof.

Improving Your Work Over Time

Feedback from others—a professor, an editor, a peer reviewer, or even a friend—provides you with essential information you can use to improve your writing. I have read more manuscripts and student papers than I care to admit, and I have noticed that most people make two or three errors over and over again when they write. Maybe they are poor spellers or use the wrong word because their vocabulary is limited. Maybe they have trouble organizing or staying on track, or maybe they use prepositions incorrectly or have trouble with parallel construction. These common errors can earn your paper or manuscript a low mark or a rejection slip. Learning to notice your most common errors and how to correct them takes a little effort but will have huge payoffs for your writing.

Make a list of the errors your reviewers find, and use it during the editing phase to catch mistakes before anyone else sees them. One of my common errors is poor spelling; for example, I can't ever recall if it's *chose* or *choose*. When in doubt, I reach for the dictionary. I still remember Evelyn Jaffe, one of my occupational therapy professors, correcting my misuse of *that* and *which;* I specifically proofread for this error. I'm also prone to run-on sentences, so my editing process will include adding periods and deleting extra words and breaking up paragraphs. Finally, I am a self-confessed slasher who is likely to write 20 pages off topic before I force myself back to task.

Following an organized outline and strong thesis statement keeps me focused on the topic at hand. Used in this way, feedback is a coveted acquisition and the most highly prized tool in your writer's toolkit, as it is the one that can catapult your writing to success.

> **Feedback is a coveted acquisition and the most highly prized tool in your writer's toolkit, as it is the one that can catapult your writing to success.**

Updating Your Writing Toolkit

Writing is a craft, honed and refined by hard work. Joy comes when you get your ideas down just as you want them and communicate to others in a way only the written word can. To practice their craft, writers need a toolkit well stocked with the basics and a structure for arranging their ideas on paper. Strengthening your toolkit, following the writing process, and sleuthing out and eliminating errors will help you refresh, renew, and remediate your writing and ultimately help you become "a writer."

REFERENCES

Ackerman, D. (1990). *A natural history of the senses*. New York: Vintage Books.

American Psychological Association. (2010). *Publication manual of the American Psychological Association* (6th ed.). Washington, DC: Author.

DeVincent-Hayes, N. (1995). *Grammar and diagramming sentences*. Eugene, OR: Garlic Press.

Dunn, W. (2008). *Living sensationally: Understanding your senses*. London: Jessica Kingsley.

Elbow, P. (2008). *Writing with power: Techniques for mastering the writing process* (2nd ed.). New York: Oxford University Press.

Emerson, R. W. (n.d.). *Columbia world of quotations*. Retrieved April 13, 2013, from Dictionary.com Web site: http://quotes.dictionary.com/We_are_as_much_informed_of_a_writers

Gibaldi, J. (2008). *MLA style manual and guide to scholarly publishing* (3rd ed.). New York: Modern Language Association of America.

Hacker, D. (2006). *A writer's reference* (6th ed.). New York: Bedford/St. Martin's.

O'Connor, P. T. (1998). *Woe is I: The grammarphobe's guide to better English in plain English*. New York: Riverhead Books.

Reilly, M. (1962). Occupational therapy can be one of the great ideas of 20th-century medicine (Eleanor Clarke Slagle Lecture). *American Journal of Occupational Therapy, 16*, 1–9.

Shortz, W. (1996). *The puzzlemaster presents: 200 mind-bending challenges from NPR*. New York: Random House.

Shortz, W. (2004). *The puzzlemaster presents: Vol. 2. Will Shortz's best puzzles from NPR*. New York: Random House.

Truss, L. (2004). *Eats, shoots and leaves: The zero tolerance approach to punctuation*. New York: Gotham Books.

Vonnegut, K. (1998). *Timequake*. New York: Berkley.

5

What Editors Wish You Knew

ROBERT G. HESS, JR., RN, PhD, FAAN, and LISA FOULKE, BA

Writing is easy; all you have to do is sit staring at a blank sheet of paper until drops of blood appear on your forehead.

—GENE FOWLER

S usan's submission was coming along fine. Her manuscript was the correct length, in the publication's style, and submitted on time. She had revised her manuscript by responding to every critique made by the editorial team and reviewers. The final version was copyedited and proofread, sent to Susan for approval, and scheduled to go to press. Susan's article would be published.

Michael's manuscript, however, was too long by 2,000 words, ignored the publication's style requirements, and was a week past deadline. His response to the managing editor about correcting these problems was, "You're the editor; just clean it up for me." The editor cleaned it up by sending Michael a rejection letter.

Why Write and Publish?

Print and online professional journals and magazines are still the primary method of disseminating new research—the lifeblood that keeps practitioners current and up to date.

Health care professionals, such as occupational therapists, write for publication for a variety of reasons. Professional obligation drives some because the hallmark of a health care profession is that its practice must be based on a unique body of evidence and knowledge. Print and online professional journals and magazines are still the primary method of disseminating new research—the lifeblood that keeps practitioners current and up to date.

Beyond disseminating research, writing for publication presents opportunities for health care professionals to tell their stories, report events and innovations, and celebrate their practice. It is a way to mold new professionals' behavior and describe what, specifically, a profession holds near and dear—the way it defines itself.

Writing for publication also holds promise for strengthening a career, building that publications section of a CV, and stroking an ego. It's a kick to get published, and some of us go back over and over again to that thrill of seeing our names associated with an article by writing one more manuscript.

Optimizing Your Opportunities to Publish

Writers who want to publish need three things—an appropriate publication, a suitable topic, and a sympathetic editor.

FINDING AN APPROPRIATE PUBLICATION

When you begin to consider writing an article, think about where you would like to publish it. The simplest way to assess whether your idea fits the content of a journal or magazine is to read or scan a year's worth of issues. Get a sense of the readership, which becomes your target audience. Get a feel for the titles and authors, the way material is written and presented, and the topics the editors have chosen to publish. Also note what's missing. Editors are always looking to provide health care professionals with information they need to know before they know they need to know it. This mantra has editors constantly scanning the environment for new topics that may soon become relevant to their own readership.

Journals and magazines that publish letters to the editor offer a quick way to get your name in print (and to be noticed by editorial staff). Editors thrive on intelligent reactions to the material they publish. Believe us, no bigger disappointment exists for an editor than to publish a hard-hitting, controversial topic and then get no reaction from the readers. It's like publishing to a dead zone, and editors wonder if there's real life out there somewhere among the readers. The quicker you react to a recently published article, the better your chances are of having your letter published. But keep your letter short and to the point. If your letter is clear, insightful, provocative, and lucky enough to be noticed, you might even evoke a response from another reader that is printed in the next issue, one of the highest forms of collegial dialogue you can hope for.

Regularly scheduled columns and departments that address clinical topics, new medications or treatment modules, or ethical and legal aspects of the profession are all opportunities to be published, if an editor allows guest entries. Some journals and magazines regularly publish book reviews, and the editor may allow you to write one, if you ask. Last, be on the lookout for upcoming special issues dedicated to certain themes, such as technology or changes in specific practice areas. Editors can become particularly needy for manuscripts if they are revisiting a topic area they address on a repeated basis.

SELECTING A SUITABLE TOPIC

Journals are generally consistent in the content they produce, so make sure your topic matches the usual content. Editors and production directors may occasionally redesign a magazine for a fresh look or deviate from customary content in response to current events or changes in practice, but by and large, editors of successful journals believe they know what content their readers want. So they deliver it over and over again.

The readers and the mission of the journal guide the editors in determining the content. For example, the *American Journal of Occupational Therapy*, an official publication of the American Occupational Therapy Association, is a peer-reviewed journal that focuses on research, practice, and health care issues in the field of occupational therapy. Manuscripts about new manual techniques for treating patients with back injuries or clinical research studies comparing techniques in invasive cardiac diagnostic procedures would probably be rejected on their titles alone unless aspects of these topics had relevance to occupational therapists. Likewise, *Today in OT,* a magazine that publishes news relevant to occupational therapists and reports clinical and career updates, would not publish original, peer-reviewed research. It's just not what that publication does.

Editors appreciate writers who can identify new trends and then provide a publishable manuscript that addresses them. They also look for articles that fill holes in the literature—areas of information that need dissemination but have somehow been missed—or that revisit subjects that have been addressed previously but need an update or that warrant another visit because you, as a creative and insightful writer, have found a new and refreshing way to present them.

Your topic should pass the following tests:

- Is the topic appropriately narrow? For example, "The challenges diabetic children face" is not as specific as "How diabetic children are discriminated against in school."
- Is the subject timely? How long a shelf life will it have?
- Is the subject realistic and manageable? Can it be summarized in a single sentence?
- Is the subject relevant? Can it pass the "So what?" and "What's new?" tests?
- Is there an audience? If so, is it the readership of the publication you're targeting?

Some professionals are simply trying to publish research from their school papers, master's theses, or doctoral dissertations. Editors know and (should) respect and expect that. As a potential author, you should be up front when attempting to publish schoolwork. If editors believe your subject matter is worthy, they can provide the best guidance about how to present your project through their publications. If you are a student or a recent graduate and you are tempted to send an unrevised student paper into a journal for publication, don't. Unsolicited (especially unaltered) school papers usually find themselves in the trash can, unread. However, do think about using previously written and carefully researched student papers as the basis for new manuscripts, but only after they are revised to the specifications of a journal and focused by direction from its editor.

CULTIVATING THE SYMPATHY OF AN EDITOR

Editors look for qualities that indicate good writing. Good writers demonstrate curiosity and attention to detail. Editors appreciate this latter characteristic because it cuts down on the inaccuracies of information found in manuscripts when they are fact-checked. Good editors will check your sources and details. An interesting manner and style and skill in using simple language to convey meaning also engage editors looking for brilliant submissions. Finally, be a hero to an editor, and steer him or her to a new, exciting topic.

Although reporting research involves formulaic components (problem, literature review, methodology, results, and discussion), boring isn't one of them. The first few sentences of any story or article—the *lead* (or *lede;* also called a *hook*) in journalist terms—are critical because they tell readers what the story is about. An editor will assess whether your lead will hook your readers and keep them reading. The following are examples of effective leads:

- Open with a question: "What's it going to be then, eh?"—Anthony Burgess, *A Clockwork Orange*
- Use sensory words—colors, textures, smells, sounds (Chalfant & Habel, 2008)—to set the scene: "In a hole in the ground there lived a hobbit. Not a nasty, dirty, wet hole, filled with the ends of worms and an oozy smell, nor yet a dry, bare, sandy hole with nothing in it to sit down on or to eat: it was a hobbit-hole, and that means comfort."—J.R.R. Tolkien, *The Hobbit*
- Shake up the reader: "Marley was dead, to begin with. There is no doubt whatever about that."—Charles Dickens, *A Christmas Carol*

MY FAVORITE LEADS

"Try doing anything without using your hands and you'll understand how patients may feel while recovering from hand tendon transfer surgery. Whether preparing a meal, getting dressed, typing, or using a mouse, having only one hand for performing tasks can be a lesson in frustration." (Williams, 2008)

"If the average age of an American nurse is 46 years, chances are that one-third of the female nurses who read this article have urinary incontinence." (Nichols, Albaugh, & Seidel, n.d.)

—Robert G. Hess, Jr., RN, PhD, FAAN

The lead should grab the reader. Look for an element of surprise, something a little quirky, jolting, or unusual; play on the unexpected. But keep it short—fewer than 35 words, even a single sentence, leading up to why the reader should care about what follows. Keep the tone of the publication in mind when crafting your lead. If you're writing for a serious medical journal, don't be too cute. If the tone of the publication is lighter, you have a little more wiggle room.

Like dance instructors partnering with their students in a pro-am competition, editors are there to make you look good. Sometimes it's as simple as moving a sentence from the body of the narrative to the beginning. Like professional dancers, they are experts at technique and style, as in word flow and the orderly progression of written thought. Some editors are writers themselves, but most have concentrated on honing the skills to enhance your writing and chances of publication.

Editors' jobs are to fill their publications with quality pieces, so they need writers. The same empty pages face them every press cycle. But editors need writers who follow rules—not only style requirements that outline the process and structure for submitting manuscripts to their particular publications but also rules of language and common courtesy (see Chapters 4, 7, and 14 in this volume).

Editors also look for the following indicators of a well-written manuscript:

- Subheadings are used to orient the readers and tie the narrative together.
- The article is focused and has a consistent point of view (i.e., voice).
- The language is succinct, and sentence lengths vary.
- The narrative is active and simple, at a seventh- or eighth-grade reading level.
- The article has practical value and targets the reader.
- Statistics and anecdotes are used judiciously.
- Ideas flow logically from one to the next, and transitions are smooth.
- Every word is necessary.
- Each issue is addressed in one place only, not several times throughout the manuscript.
- The introduction clearly states what the article is about, and the content of the article matches the introduction.
- The conclusion refers back to and carries forward the introduction, indicating the writer has remained focused on his or her clearly stated purpose.

- It (almost) goes without saying that the author has used good grammar, spot-on spelling, wise word choices, and proper punctuation (specifics are covered in Chapter 4 in this volume).

The Publishing Process

The sections that follow describe the publishing process for peer-reviewed and non-peer-reviewed publications. The differences between them are noted as appropriate.

WRITER'S GUIDELINES AND STYLE GUIDES

Writer's guidelines are a set of instructions put together by a publication that specify its requirements for material from writers. Read them carefully. Editors are swamped with submissions from writers who never bother to read either the publication or its writer's guidelines. Some editors refuse even to read submissions that are not written in their publication's style. The guidelines should list the sections of the publication that feature unsolicited manuscripts; preferred format, style, and length; and whether and how much the publisher pays.

A *style guide* is a set of standards for writing that details everything from how to spell certain words (e.g., is *health care* one word or two?) to how to properly reference a source (e.g., in a footnote? author–date citation?). This book uses the sixth edition of the *Publication Manual of the American Psychological Association* (American Psychological Association, 2010) as well as several pages of style rules particular to this publisher.

QUERY LETTERS AND CALLS

If you are submitting to a magazine (peer-reviewed journals generally accept only completed manuscripts), contact the editor before you start writing to see if he or she is interested in an article on your chosen topic. By contacting the editor before writing, you can easily avoid submitting a manuscript that does not fit with the journal or that deals with a topic that has been previously published or will be covered by an already accepted manuscript. It pays to do your homework. Look for the editor's contact information in the magazine's masthead or on its Web site. Don't be afraid

> By contacting the editor before writing, you can easily avoid submitting a manuscript that does not fit with the journal or that deals with a topic that has been previously published or will be covered by an already accepted manuscript.

to pick up the phone. Some of the most prestigious editors are amazingly accessible by phone or e-mail, and they'll let you know how they like to be contacted. You should also take the opportunity to ask for a copy of the guidelines and find out which style guide the publication uses.

If you write a query letter or e-mail, be sure to craft it carefully to entice the editor with your topic idea. This is a time to show your creativity and expertise and to demonstrate that you can write. If you are addressing a clinical topic, establish why you are qualified to write about the topic by including your credentials and relevant experience. Don't send or attach a résumé or CV at this point; just justify your qualification to write about your topic. Succinctly explain your article idea: for example, "I'd like to do a continuing education module on distal radius fractures that details risk factors, treatments through the healing processes, and complications."

Your query should be structured like a business letter and written on appropriate stationery or in a formal business e-mail. If you have professional letterhead, use it. If you're sending an e-mail, use your professional electronic signature. Address the letter to a specific editor using the editor's correctly spelled name, gender, title, and credentials. Have someone other than yourself proof the document before sending.

TENTATIVE ACCEPTANCE

After submitting a manuscript to a journal or magazine, you get to wait for the verdict from the editor. You should make sure your work was actually received, so feel free to send a follow-up letter or e-mail if no acknowledgment is forthcoming. Some publications' writer's guidelines provide a time frame that lets you know when to expect an acknowledgment that your manuscript has been received. If not, wait a week and follow up. Be persistent if you don't hear back in a week or so. (Submissions made electronically may receive an immediate e-mail acknowledgment.) If your query is favorably received, you should expect clarification from the editor about the overall process and finer details to guide your writing, deadlines, and manuscript length.

ACCEPTANCE AND REVIEW

Acceptance of a manuscript submitted to a magazine is a tentative status that usually becomes finalized only when the manuscript is ready for publication. When a manuscript is initially accepted, expect a long process of rewriting and revising in response to comments from editors and reviewers. Some exceptional submissions are reviewed and accepted with hardly a change in commas, but most undergo some level of revision. An editor accepts or rejects a manuscript on the basis of his or her experience. Either the editor or a managing editor guides the revision process and helps you refine your manuscript for publication. You can expect your editor's respect and expertise. In return, you should also do everything you can to be respectful of the editorial process.

When a manuscript is initially accepted, expect a long process of rewriting and revising in response to comments from editors and reviewers.

When a manuscript is submitted to a peer-reviewed journal, an editor reviews it and decides whether to send it to experts who critique the content. The experts may occasionally edit, but their job is to assess the quality and currency of the content, point out any factual errors, and make recommendations for improvement. To reduce the potential for bias, the process is usually blinded, so the reviewers don't know who the authors are and vice versa. The quality of many articles depends on the quality of the reviewers, so the editor must choose well. Some editors use reviewers from an editorial board who are experts in the general subject area, and others select reviewers on the basis of the specific, circumscribed expertise.

Selection of reviewers is a serious process. Choosing the wrong reviewer, one who is inexperienced in reviewing or even an expert whose knowledge is incomplete or out of date, can lead to publication of manuscripts that are outside the purview of the publication or that have inaccuracies or omissions. Reviewers come with a variety of experience as reviewers and corresponding levels of tact. Good reviewers usually have had their own work reviewed by others and offer valuable critique. You should be responsive to authentic critique and disregard criticism that borders on personal attack. Editors try to winnow out the latter, but if they don't, focus on your manuscript and move on. Remember, regardless of the reviewers' verdicts, the editor makes the decision for acceptance or rejection.

DEADLINES

Peer-reviewed or not, track the progress of your manuscript by staying in touch with the editor through whatever means he or she prefers (many publishers have electronic submission systems that send acknowledgment at predetermined times throughout the process). Editors have their own time frames set by peer review, their customary editorial process, and a publishing schedule. Soon after they have accepted your article, they will schedule a tentative publication date. Editors have a seemingly endless amount of blank pages that they must fill, over and over again. Because they depend on a predictable flow of publishable manuscripts, the deadlines they set with writers and reviewers are sacrosanct.

Don't ever ignore a deadline. Editors have incredible memories when it comes to being burned by writers who miss deadlines. You might have to negotiate a deadline, but don't ever ignore one.

REJECTION

If your manuscript is rejected, be sure to find out why. Was the content not appropriate? Was the writing or manuscript preparation inadequate? You have an opportunity to learn at this point, if you have a willing editor. Try to take advantage of this, and find out if the rejection is negotiable. Maybe the editor is willing to read another submission with revisions.

Remember that everyone who decides to share his or her words with someone else will eventually get a rejection letter. Talent does not guarantee

---

FIRST PUBLICATIONS

My first peer-reviewed article was published in a journal that had rejected my dozen previous attempts. The editor called me and said, "Bob, if you could just write your manuscript like you write your query letters, we'd publish your work." She encouraged a consultation with a member of her editorial advisory board who advised me to avoid *"orgo-babble"*—a coined, technical term for obtuse, meaningless, academic-sounding bad writing. After a favorable review and a strong edit, I was published in a professional journal.

—*Robert G. Hess, Jr., RN, PhD, FAAN*

publication. Editors have rejected many now-famous books (Bernard, 1990)—for example:

- *The Diary of Anne Frank*—"The girl doesn't, it seems to me, have a special perception or feeling which would lift that book above the curiosity level."
- *Catch-22*, by Joseph Heller—"A continual and unmitigated bore."
- *Animal Farm,* by George Orwell—"It is impossible to sell animal stories in the U.S.A."

Keeping Editors on Your Side

Writing is fun and tedious, but a big payoff awaits those who learn the craft and successfully publish. The personal and professional satisfaction of seeing your work in print or online is hard to beat. Know that you have company as you soldier on through hours of writing and deliberation. We editors will be with you in spirit as we whack away at our own manuscripts.

REFERENCES

American Psychological Association. (2010). *Publication manual of the American Psychological Association* (6th ed.). Washington, DC: Author.

Bernard, A. (1990). *Rotten rejections: A literary companion.* New York: Pushcart Press.

Chalfant, A., & Habel, M. (2008). *Writing well: A nurse's handbook* [Continuing education course]. Hoffman Estates, IL: Gannett Healthcare Group.

Nichols, A., Albaugh, J., & Seidel, S. L. (n.d.). *The management of urinary incontinence* [Continuing education course]. Hoffman Estates, IL: Gannett Healthcare Group. Retrieved March 21, 2012, from http://ce.nurse.com/ce128-60/the-management-of-urinary-incontinence

Williams, S. (2008). Hand in hand. *Today in OT.* Retrieved March 21, 2012, from http://news.todayinot.com/article/20080929/TODAYINOT010303/80926003&SearchID=73458335128947

BOOKS EDITORS WISH YOU WOULD READ

Alward, E. C., & Alward, J. A. (1997). *Punctuation plain and simple.* Pompton Plains, NJ: Career Press.

Dupré, L. (1995). *BUGS in writing: A guide to debugging your prose.* Reading, MA: Addison-Wesley Professional.

Eggenschwiller, J., & Dotson, E. (2001). *CliffsQuickReview™ writing: Grammar, usage, and style.* New York: Wiley.

Hale, C. (1999). *Sin and syntax.* New York: Broadway Books.

Lamott, A. (1994). *Bird by bird: Some instructions on writing and life.* New York: Doubleday.

Lederer, R. (1999). *Sleeping dogs don't lay.* New York: St. Martin's.

Saver, C. (2011). *Anatomy of writing for publication for nurses.* Indianapolis, IN: Sigma Theta Tau International.

Strunk, W., Jr., & White, E. B. (1999). *The elements of style* (4th ed.). Upper Saddle River, NJ: Pearson Education.

Taggart, C., & Wines, J. A. (2009). *My grammar and I (or should that be "me"?): Old-school ways to sharpen your English.* Pleasantville, NY: Reader's Digest Association.

Tracz, R. F. (1991). *Dr. Grammar's writes from wrongs: A supremely authoritative guide to the common and not-so-common rules of the English language.* New York: Vintage Books.

Truss, L. (2003). *Eats, shoots and leaves: The zero tolerance approach to punctuation.* New York: Gotham Books.

Zinsser, W. (1990). *On writing well: An informal guide to writing nonfiction* (4th ed.). New York: Harper Perennial.

RESOURCES TO HONE YOUR WRITING SKILLS

Hiemstra, R. (2007). *Tips for greater success in writing journal articles.* Retrieved March 21, 2012, from http://www-distance.syr.edu/writingtips.html

Pollard, R. Q., Jr. (2005). From dissertation to journal article: A useful method for planning and writing any manuscript. *Internet Journal of Mental Health, 2*(2). Retrieved March 21, 2012, from http://www.ispub.com/ostia/index.php?xml FilePath=journals/ijmh/vol2n2/writing.xml

Science Fiction and Fantasy Writers of America. (n.d.). *Writers beware: Warnings about the schemes, scams, and pitfalls that threaten writers.* Retrieved March 21, 2012, from http://www.sfwa.org/for-authors/writer-beware

Sharp, C. (2000). *A writer's workbook: Daily exercises for the writing life.* New York: St. Martin's.

Sherrill, C. D. (2003). *Writing journal articles.* Retrieved March 21, 2012, from http://vergil.chemistry.gatech.edu/resources/writing-papers.pdf

Poets & Writers: http://www.pw.org

Resources for Writers: http://resourcesforwriters.suite101.com

University of Maine Writing Center: http://www.umaine.edu/wcenter/resources

Writing Corner: http://writingcorner.com

Writing-World: http://www.writing-world.com

6

What You Should Know About Collaboration and Copyright

SHARON A. GUTMAN, PhD, OTR, FAOTA

In the short term, we always overstate the effects of new technologies. But in the long run, we always underestimate them.
—RICHARD THIEME (AS CITED IN VEEN & VRAKKING, 2006)

Collaborative writing can be one of the most creative and stimulating processes in an academic career. Sharing ideas, jointly transforming ideas into a tangible product, and disseminating collaboratively developed work to the scholarly community provide a wealth of opportunities to develop new skills and grow professionally. Collaboration is one of the best ways to challenge yourself to learn about novel information, think beyond your comfort zone, and master skills that once seemed beyond your reach.

Collaborating as part of an interdisciplinary team of authors provides you with the opportunity to learn from another profession's body of knowledge, benefit from resources across professions, and enhance other health professionals' knowledge about occupational therapy. Many grant funders seek and favor interdisciplinary teamwork on research and practice projects. The resources needed to complete most research studies are beyond the reach of one person alone, but a team of professionals who each offers a highly specialized skill set and access to varying resources is better able to develop and complete specific projects.

Although collaboration is essential for scholars and researchers, success in joint efforts requires an awareness of the problems that may arise in the collaborative process—from the birth of an idea to publication and copyright. Knowledge of the risks is essential to prevent possible harm to the parties involved. This chapter describes challenges inherent in collaborative writing and effective ways to anticipate these challenges, provides an overview of copyright practices, and discusses issues in negotiating fair publication contracts.

Authorship

Once you and your colleagues begin discussing a specific writing project and invite potential coauthors to participate, you should also discuss who will appear as authors in the final product. According to the *Publication Manual of the American Psychological Association* (American Psychological Association, 2010), *authors* are those who have made a substantial contribution to a published work by doing one or more of the following: writing large sections of the manuscript or the manuscript in full, generating the idea for the project and supervising the steps needed for completion, participating in large portions of intervention provision and data collection, or conducting the statistical analysis and interpreting the results. Anyone who has made a lesser contribution should be noted in an acknowledgment section. Lesser contributions include providing advice or guidance about the study (e.g., related to research design, methodological procedures, statistical analysis), recruiting participants, participating in portions of intervention provision and data collection, and entering data and managing databases.

> *Authors* are those who have made a substantial contribution to a published work by . . . writing large sections of the manuscript or the manuscript in full, generating the idea for the project and supervising the steps needed for completion, participating in large portions of intervention provision and data collection, or conducting the statistical analysis and interpreting the results.

AUTHORSHIP ORDER

Your discussion of authorship in the early stages of a writing project should specify the order of authors, with the understanding that the order may change as the project evolves and anticipated contributions change or are modified. The principal contributor to a writing project or research study is listed as first author, and subsequent authors are typically listed in order of decreasing level of contribution.

Any decisions you and your team make during initial project discussions about who will appear as authors and in what order should be recorded in writing, along with the date and names of those present for each discussion. If project members' roles and contributions change unexpectedly over time, your group should renegotiate authorship and rerecord your agreement. It is also good practice for the team leader or a designated member to document each person's role in a project, specifying the precise activities associated with that role and timelines and due dates for each step of the assigned activities.

All project members should receive, review, and sign copies of meeting notes, documents listing anticipated authorship and order, and descriptions of team members' roles. Having team members sign these documents can prevent delays in publication caused by later claims to authorship by team members who do not fulfill their role expectations.

STUDENT PARTICIPATION

Occupational therapy students often participate in research under the mentorship of faculty members to begin to acquire the skills of scholarship and research. As in other projects, authorship is established on the basis of the students' contribution to the project. When faculty members supervising students generate the research question or take the lead in revising the written manuscript to meet publication standards, those faculty members should be listed first as authors. Doctoral students are expected to generate their own original work under the mentorship of an academic committee; when they turn their work into a journal article or book, they are credited as first author and doctoral committee members as coauthors, again depending on the level of contribution.

Graduate students who participate in faculty-generated research are not entitled to publish the data as their own, and again, it is important to clarify, in writing, expectations about student roles in the project and whether such roles merit coauthorship or acknowledgment. It is good practice for occupational therapy programs to ask students to sign releases before working on faculty-originated research projects. Such releases make it clear to students that data collected in the course of their education—when faculty originated—rightfully belong to the faculty mentor. For example, the Programs in Occupational Therapy at Columbia University require students to sign the following release statement before participating in faculty-originated research:

> Students enrolled in Columbia University's Programs in Occupational Therapy are required to participate with faculty in the conduct of research studies. Students are required to deliver to the Occupational Therapy Program all records, notes, data, drafts, and other materials in the student's possession regarding such research studies. Whenever requested by the Occupational Therapy Program, students will execute documentation of such delivery and related conveyance of rights. (Columbia University Programs in Occupational Therapy, 2010)

Faculty mentors may wish to wait until they have substantially revised the manuscript for publication before offering authorship to students who worked on the project. Student performance cannot be predicted before completion of a research project; if students' contribution to the project is substantially inferior to faculty expectations, an acknowledgment may be more appropriate than authorship. Once the manuscript is finalized, the faculty mentor can designate students as coauthors and contact them to obtain their agreement and consent.

FIRST-AUTHOR RESPONSIBILITIES

The person designated as first author is often responsible for making sure that the project runs smoothly and is completed on time. This may entail assuming roles that other project members cannot fulfill or finding replacements to fill those roles. When preparing a manuscript for publication, the first author is responsible for the following activities:

- Obtaining author guidelines and making sure that the manuscript adheres to the publisher's style guidelines and to its requirements relating to formatting, word count, and figure and table count
- Editing the manuscript for spelling, grammar, and punctuation errors
- Responding to reviewer comments, making requested revisions, and resubmitting the manuscript in a timely manner
- Making sure that all coauthor release forms are submitted to the publisher if the paper is accepted
- For journal articles, selecting one or more appropriate journals to submit to.

First authors typically are also responsible for obtaining permission to reprint or adapt copyrighted material from other sources, as described in the next section.

Respecting the Copyright of Others

Before reprinting copyrighted work (i.e., work that is not in the public domain) in your own work or photocopying and distributing such work, in part or in full, you must seek written permission from the copyright owner. An online version of a work will generally provide the copyright holder's identity. In a request for permission you should do the following (Columbia University Copyright Advisory Office, 2009b):

1. State your name, credentials, and academic position or employment.
2. Identify the exact information you are seeking permission to use. Indicate if you wish to use the entire work or a specific section (e.g., specific page numbers). It is good practice to provide a photocopy of the exact material you wish to use and to include the citation of the source of the material.
3. Describe how you intend to use the work. For example, indicate if your use is commercial or nonprofit, for education, or for research and publication.
4. Indicate the length of time you wish to use the work. For example, you may wish to photocopy and distribute a specific journal article in one of your classes in a given semester of a specific year.
5. State how the work will be used. For example, indicate if the work will be used in a textbook for occupational therapy students, placed in a course pack for occupational therapy students in a specific semester of a specific year, or posted to a password-protected online course repository for occupational therapy students during a specific semester of a specific year.

Box 6.1 provides a sample permission request letter.

Protecting Your Copyright

The U.S. Copyright Act grants automatic copyright ownership to authors of an original work expressed in a fixed medium (such as writing) and does not require any action from the author, such as copyright registration (U.S. Copyright Office, 2009). *Copyright* is "a form of protection grounded in the

BOX 6.1.

EXAMPLE OF A LETTER REQUESTING PERMISSION TO REPRINT COPYRIGHTED MATERIAL

[Date]

Dear Dr. Jones,

My name is Dolores Smith, PhD, OTR, and I am an associate professor in the Department of Occupational Therapy at Chesapeake University. I am writing a textbook for occupational therapy students on the cognitive assessment of neurologically impaired patients. In my data searches, I located your scale on your personal Web site at http://jones.cognitivescale.com.

I am contacting you to seek permission to reprint your scale in full in the following textbook, which is currently in preparation:

Smith, D. (in press). *Cognitive screening of patients with neurological impairment: An instruction manual for occupational therapists.* [Location]: [Publisher].

If you grant me permission to reprint your scale, your name will appear in a footnote to the scale as the copyright holder, along with a statement indicating you have granted permission for the one-time reprinting of your scale in the first edition of my book.

If you do not own the copyright to this scale, please provide any information you might have regarding the current copyright holder. Otherwise, your permission confirms that you are the rightful copyright owner and hold the right to grant the requested permission.

If you would like additional information, please feel free to contact me at the Chesapeake University Department of Occupational Therapy, Chesapeake, VA 23320; dsmith@chesapeake.edu.

I have enclosed a duplicate copy of this permission request for your own records. If you grant permission to reprint as described above, please sign this letter where noted below, and mail one copy back to me in the enclosed self-addressed, stamped envelope.

I greatly appreciate your help. Thank you for your consideration.

Sincerely,
[signature]
Dolores Smith, PhD, OTR

I grant permission for the use of the requested material as described above:

_____   _____
David D. Jones, MD, PhD   Date

U.S. Constitution and granted by law for original works of authorship fixed in a tangible medium of expression" (U.S. Copyright Office, 2006).

NEGOTIATING COPYRIGHT WITH COAUTHORS

Although copyright ownership is straightforward when only one author is involved, it is less clear when a group of authors is credited with authorship. Copyright ownership is most important for work that has the potential to generate profits (e.g., sales from books, clinical assessments, continuing education course materials). When two or more scholars have authored a work that might generate profits, they must negotiate the details of the copyright agreement in the early project stages to ensure that the division of royalties and the right to use and be credited for derivative work are fair and transparent.

All authors must agree in advance whether they will receive an equal royalty percentage or whether royalties will be distributed according to contribution level (see Chapter 14 in this volume for more information). Once the authors have made that determination, they can sign a publisher's agreement or contract stipulating those terms.

Derivative works include scholarship based on the original work, as well as translations, revisions, or other adaptations (University of Chicago Press, 2010). Authors readying a work for publication should be aware of the potential for derivative work and negotiate contracts that protect all coauthors by allowing them to maintain credit and royalties from future use of the original work. For example, two authors wrote a book, and several years later the publisher requested a second edition (the derivative work). The first author could not participate in the preparation of the second edition because of other obligations. The original second author agreed to write the second edition and was legally able to use much of the material from the first edition without crediting the original first author because the copyright belonged to the publisher. The first author lost both author credit and the ability to earn royalties from the original work.

NEGOTIATING COPYRIGHT WITH PUBLISHERS

Fair copyright contracts allow authors to retain the right to use their work in future scholarship and for educational purposes, to control the future use of their work, and to facilitate access to their work by members of the scholarly community (Columbia University Copyright Advisory Office, 2009a; Crews, 1993, 2001). Before you negotiate a copyright contract with a publisher, it is important to anticipate your future needs associated with your scholarship. The following are the most common needs and rights scholars have for their work following publication (Crews, 1993, 2001):

> **Before you negotiate a copyright contract with a publisher, it is important to anticipate your future needs associated with your scholarship.**

- Need to reproduce and distribute the work in teaching
- Need to reprint sections of the work in future articles or books
- Right to create related or derivative work (journal articles, books, professional presentations)
- Right to be credited as author of original work that has been released in another form
- Right to receive royalties for profit-generating work that has been released in another form
- Right to post journal articles (in preprint or postprint form) to their university's digital repository
- Right to post federally funded journal article research (in preprint or postprint form) to federal digital repositories in accordance with government policies.

Many publishers allow authors to negotiate copyright contracts consistent with these needs. SHERPA is a nonprofit online service (http://www.sherpa. ac.uk) whose mission is to inform the public about copyright and online archiving (SHERPA, 2006a). RoMEO, a subsidiary service of SHERPA, provides information to the public about the copyright policies of all publishers. Authors can use the RoMEO system to identify publishers whose copyright agreements provide the fairest and most liberal retention of author rights (SHERPA, 2006c).

Unless authors are vigilant in ensuring that copyright contracts treat their needs fairly, they may lose control over the rights to their own work. The following are examples of contract issues that may lead to problems (Columbia University Scholarly Communication Program, 2009):

1. *A requirement to pay to use your own work:* The contract should give authors the right to use their own work. Such a provision would exclude

authors from the requirement to seek permission and to pay to reprint a clinical scale they developed or to use their own journal article in teaching a class.

2. *Failure to preserve author credit and royalties from derivative work:* The contract should specify that if derivative works are developed using the original work of the authors, the original authors will be credited and are entitled to royalties.

3. *Loss of control over the release of outdated scholarship:* The contract should specify that if the work becomes outdated, the publisher is not authorized to continue distributing it. For example, a scholar published practice guidelines for neurodevelopmental intervention with people who have experienced traumatic brain injury (TBI). Five years later, the same scholar substantially modified the original practice guidelines on the basis of research and intervention outcomes, and she could no longer support the use of the originally published guidelines. Unless the contract specified otherwise, the publisher would be legally able to reprint the original practice guidelines in a newly released book about TBI interventions. Even if the author were credited, her name would be associated with outdated clinical information that she no longer supported.

When to Retain Copyright

In some instances, it is beneficial to authors to retain copyright and grant permission for the one-time printing of the work in a particular journal article or book. For example, authors of clinical assessments, clinical protocols, and diagnostic scales who wish to publish such materials within the body of a journal article or book should retain the copyright of such materials and grant one-time permission to print the work in a specific publication. Many publishers concur with the author retaining copyright in these instances.

Similarly, if authors have developed unique figures (e.g., illustrations, photographs, flow charts) that they wish to use again in future publications or education, they should retain the copyright of such materials and grant one-time permission to print. Retaining copyright allows authors to preserve control of specified materials and eliminates situations in which authors must seek permission and pay for future use of their own work.

Out-of-Print Clauses

Book publishing contracts often include an out-of-print clause. Publishers should have exclusive rights to a work only during the time they are actively marketing and selling the book—in other words, while the book is in print. When the book goes out of print and no longer generates a profit, the out-of-print clause allows the authors to terminate the contract and regain all rights originally transferred to the publisher. Authors can then regain control over that material and remarket it. This right is particularly important when authors believe that their work has greater potential appeal but was not adequately marketed by the publisher.

The contract must clearly define the term *out of print*—for example, a specified minimum number of books sold in a specified time period (Keep Your Copyrights & Trustees of Columbia University, 2010). This definition has become particularly important because digital media now enable publishers to print books on demand. Some publishers have argued that, because of digital on-demand publishing, books never go out of print (Authors Guild, 2010). Authors should be aware of both the need for an out-of-print clause and the need to define *out of print* using minimum sales in a specified time period.

Retain All Copyright Contracts

It is incumbent on authors to retain all copyright contracts and not depend on publishers to do so. Over time, as publishing houses are bought and sold, become subsidiaries of larger parent companies, and experience employee turnover, copyright contracts are easily lost. If authors do not retain a copy of their contract and their work is published in a journal or book now owned by another publisher, the author may find that he or she is legally bound by the copyright terms of the current publisher's copyright agreement. Fighting this situation in a lawsuit will likely involve a considerable investment of time and money.

Box 6.2 contains a checklist of items to consider when negotiating copyright with coauthors and publishers.

Copyright in the Digital Age

The Internet has provided access to a wealth of knowledge and information sharing. Although such access has offered immeasurable societal benefits, it has also multiplied the ways in which the rights of authors of original work can be violated. The following scenarios have unfortunately become common:

- An expert on cognitive interventions for patients with stroke attended a course on her specialty topic at a national conference. She was surprised

BOX 6.2.

CHECKLIST OF ITEMS TO NEGOTIATE WITH COAUTHORS AND PUBLISHERS

Coauthors

It is good practice to record answers to the following questions in writing and to ask all members of a project team to review and sign the documents:

- Who will be listed as an author?
- In what order will author names be listed?
- What roles will each coauthor have, and what are the precise activities of those roles? By what date must each activity be completed?
- If a work with multiple authors is potentially profit-generating, how will royalties be divided—equally or by contribution level?
- If a work has multiple authors, will all authors be credited with authorship if a derivative of the original work is generated?

Publishers

When negotiating copyright agreements with publishers, consider preserving for yourself the following rights:

- To reproduce and distribute your work for educational purposes
- To reprint sections of your work in future articles or books without needing to seek permission or pay a fee
- To create related or derivative work from your original work (e.g., course materials, continuing education workshop materials, Web sites, professional presentations, journal articles, books)
- To decide whether the publisher can release your original work in another form
- To be credited as author of the original work if it will be released in another form
- To receive royalties for profit-generating work that is released in another form
- To deposit journal articles to your university repository
- To post federally funded research to online repositories in accordance with government policies
- To define *out of print* as a specified number of sales in a specified time period.

to see the course presenter using her own PowerPoint slides verbatim without credit. The scholar thought of two ways the course presenter could have accessed her slides: (1) The slides were posted on her university course repository, and (2) she frequently presented her work to large audiences and downloaded her slides before each presentation onto the presenting facility's computer, from which anyone could download the slides onto a portable drive.

- A colleague notified a scholar that a practitioner had turned material from one of his book chapters into a continuing education workshop. The practitioner used material from the book chapter verbatim—including text, photographs, illustrations, and scales—all without credit to the author or permission from the publisher. The practitioner not only violated copyright but also used the scholar's material for her own profit—legally referred to as *bad faith use.*
- A college professor who taught in an occupational therapy program developed a screening instrument to measure cognitive status in adults with brain injury through the evaluation of a meal preparation task. The screening had not been published but was posted on her academic program's Web site. About a year after her screening was posted online, the college professor read a journal article about the development of a similar screening instrument whose authors had used items from her screening verbatim without crediting her.

New technologies—online repositories, electronic journals and books, wikispaces, blogs—have challenged traditional copyright conventions, and laws guiding copyright have not kept pace with rapidly changing publishing technologies. Nevertheless, when posting original scholarship using online technologies, authors can take certain steps to encourage users to respect their rights.

STEPS YOU CAN TAKE TO PROTECT YOUR WORK

Although U.S. copyright law does not require authors to register copyright, it is good practice to do so, particularly if the work might generate profits (e.g., clinical instruments, materials for continuing education courses). Authors should register copyright within 3 months of completing the work (Columbia University Copyright Advisory Office, 2009a). Copyright registration can be completed online for a minimal fee at www.copyright.gov. Copyright registration makes it possible to seek statutory damages in a copyright infringement case.

> **Authors who post any type of scholarship online should place a copyright notice on all work.**

Authors who post any type of scholarship online should place a copyright notice on all work. The following materials should have copyright notices: unpublished manuscripts, PowerPoint lecture slides, course notes, continuing education materials, newly developed clinical screens and evaluations, and clinical practice guidelines. A copyright notice involves three elements:

- The word "copyright" and the symbol ©
- The year the work was created
- The name of the copyright owner.

Additionally, the authors should provide contact information (e.g., an e-mail address or Web site URL) to enable others to seek permission to use the material (Keep Your Copyrights & Trustees of Columbia University, 2010). A sample copyright notice is "Copyright © 2013 by Dolores Smith, PhD, OTR. dsmith@chesapeake.edu."

If the work is intended to be shared freely for nonprofit educational and clinical use, the authors may also place a permission notice on their work to eliminate the need to contact the author. For example,

> Copyright © 2013 by Dolores Smith, PhD, OTR. dsmith@chesapeake.edu. Permission is hereby granted to reproduce and distribute copies of this work for nonprofit educational purposes, provided that copies are distributed at or below cost and that the author and copyright notice are included on each copy. (Columbia University Copyright Advisory Office, 2009c)

Using a Creative Commons license is one of the most efficient ways to grant automatic permission within specified limitations. Creative Commons is a nonprofit organization offering six standard licenses that grant varying degrees of permission; authors can license their work freely or with conditions to the public domain (Creative Commons, 2010). Creative Commons services can be accessed online at http://creativecommons.org/about/licenses.

If the authors post a work online and do not intend it to be copied or distributed without their permission, a restriction of use statement may be warranted:

> Copyright © 2013 by Dolores Smith, PhD, OTR. dsmith@chesapeake.edu. This work cannot be copied, distributed, or altered in any way without written permission from the author. Use of this work in any way other than as intended is an infringement of copyright law and is subject to penalty.

Although placing permission and restriction-of-use statements on all unpublished work intended for Internet posting is good practice, such practices alone may not be sufficient to secure damages in a copyright infringement case (Keep Your Copyrights & Trustees of Columbia University, 2010).

ONLINE TECHNOLOGIES FACILITATING ACCESS TO SCHOLARSHIP

With the abundance of online media, online systems have been developed to facilitate the sharing of scholarship and mitigate the potential for copyright violation of authors' work. Although no system can fully eradicate potential unethical uses of work, online systems of scholarship reach such a broad audience that plagiarism is recognized and exposed at a higher rate (Columbia University Copyright Advisory Office, 2009a; SHERPA, 2006b).

Open Access

The term *open access* refers to the ability to freely access scholarship using an Internet connection. Articles placed in open access venues reach far greater audiences than do articles in which the full text is restricted to subscribers. Open access articles have more readers and are cited more often in the literature than are traditionally accessed articles (Columbia University Copyright Advisory Office, 2009a; SHERPA, 2006b). Because work posted to open access venues can reach vast audiences, plagiarism is more likely to be exposed.

Open Access Journals

Open access journals provide free access to their articles by charging authors a fee before publication that covers expenses such as peer review, manuscript preparation and typesetting, and server space. (Publication expenses for traditional journals are paid through user subscriptions.) In this way stakeholders interested in the dissemination of the journal's research pay for production expenses, allowing access to the public without charge. Sometimes the research funder pays author fees; otherwise, the researcher or the researcher's academic institution must absorb publication costs. Before open access journals, most journals used a publication model in which fees were paid for after publication through subscriptions. Open access journals follow the usual peer review process and thus maintain the same level of quality as subscription-funded journals (Columbia University Copyright Advisory Office, 2009a; SHERPA, 2006b).

Open Access Repositories

Open access repositories archive digital copies or preprint versions of published articles allowing them to be freely accessed by anyone with an Internet connection. Many open access repositories are discipline specific. Before depositing materials to an open access repository, authors must confirm that their copyright agreement allows their published article to be archived. Some publishers readily allow duplicate versions of published articles, whereas others allow only preprint versions; the repository system labels the archived article as preprint or postprint. Preprint versions may contain supplemental materials that are not available in the published article. Available evidence suggests that archiving published materials in open access repositories does not affect journal subscriptions, but the open access repository system has not existed long enough to yield sufficient data to draw a firm conclusion. Nevertheless, academic communities and stakeholders who understand the importance of freely sharing knowledge are increasingly embracing open access systems (Columbia University Copyright Advisory Office, 2009a; SHERPA, 2006b).

University Repositories

Most universities have their own repositories and require faculty to deposit their publications for public access. Because of this emerging academic demand, many publishers' copyright agreements allow authors to archive their published work in their university repositories (Columbia University Copyright Advisory Office, 2009a; SHERPA, 2006b).

Funder Guidelines for Posting Published Work

In recognition of the importance of sharing research results with the scientific community and public, many funders now require authors to deposit grant-funded research articles in online repositories. For example, researchers whose work has been funded by the National Institutes of Health are required by law to post their studies in PubMed Central (Columbia University Copyright Advisory Office, 2009a; SHERPA, 2006b). Publishers whose copyright agreement does not recognize this requirement are out of compliance with federal law.

Online technologies have both emerged from and strengthened the demand for open access to scholarship and the free sharing of knowledge. The demand for open access has changed traditional copyright conventions. Today, publishers that do not allow authors to deposit their scholarship to online repositories to facilitate open access are seen as outdated and restrictive. Authors are increasingly encouraged to seek publisher and copyright agreements that facilitate the sharing of their work with the scholarly community.

> **Today, publishers that do not allow authors to deposit their scholarship to online repositories to facilitate open access are seen as outdated and restrictive.**

Online open access systems self-regulate author exploitation and plagiarism through user vigilance, but self-regulation is less feasible in personal Web sites, wikispaces, blogs, and university course Web sites that are not secure because they are not as widely accessed. Posting scholarship to nonsecure online systems is inadvisable.

Protecting Your Work

Producing and disseminating original work is an integral component of the role of a scholar and is necessary to the success of an academic career. Today, collaborative work is often necessary to bring together the multiple skills and resources essential to the generation of research that can truly benefit society. The transfer of copyright ownership that occurs in the traditional publication process has always held the potential for author exploitation, especially when multiple coauthors are involved.

The ease of accessing and copying information afforded by the Internet has exponentially increased the potential for copyright violation and author harm. Yet, more than at any other time in our history, academia has recognized and called on publishers to create fair copyright agreements that protect scholars and their work. In response to academia's call, the publishing world has listened, and an increasing number of publishers now use copyright agreements that grant more liberal rights to scholars. Similarly, as the potential copyright perils of nonsecure Internet postings are recognized, the academic world has responded by endorsing vast open access systems through which plagiarism is monitored and exposed by members of the scholarly community.

Although no one mechanism can eliminate the potential for plagiarism and copyright infringement, authors who are aware of potential concerns and adopt strategies to limit their occurrence can better avoid exploitation and harm. The information contained in this chapter is basic, and authors are encouraged to seek further information and clarification about specific situations from the legal counsel at their universities and other settings.

REFERENCES

American Psychological Association. (2010). *Publication manual of the American Psychological Association* (6th ed.). Washington, DC: Author.

Authors Guild. (2010). *Improving your book contract: Negotiation tips for nine typical clauses.* Retrieved October 6, 2011, from http://www.authorsguild.org/services/legal_services/books.html

Columbia University Copyright Advisory Office. (2009a). *Copyright ownership.* Retrieved October 6, 2011, from http://copyright.columbia.edu/copyright/copyright-ownership

Columbia University Copyright Advisory Office. (2009b). *Permissions.* Retrieved October 6, 2011, from http://copyright.columbia.edu/copyright/permissions/

Columbia University Copyright Advisory Office. (2009c). *Your copyrights: Determining who owns the copyright.* Retrieved October 6, 2011, from http://copyright.columbia.edu/copyright/copyright-ownership/your-copyrights/

Columbia University Programs in Occupational Therapy. (2010). *Research release statement for entry-level occupational therapy students.* New York: Author.

Columbia University Scholarly Communication Program. (2009). *Manage your copyrights.* Retrieved October 6, 2011, from http://scholcomm.columbia.edu/manage-your-copyrights

Creative Commons. (2010). *License your work.* Retrieved October 6, 2011, from http://creativecommons.org/choose/

Crews, K. D. (1993). *Copyright, fair use, and the challenge for universities: Promoting the progress of higher education.* Chicago: University of Chicago Press.

Crews, K. D. (2001). The law of fair use and the illusion of fair-use guidelines. *Ohio State Law Journal, 62,* 602–700. Retrieved October 6, 2011, from http://moritzlaw.osu.edu/lawjournal/issues/volume62/number2/crews.pdf

Keep Your Copyrights & Trustees of Columbia University. (2010). *"Out of print" clauses.* Retrieved October 6, 2011, from http://keepyourcopyrights.org/copyright/reversion/out-of-print

SHERPA. (2006a). *About SHERPA: Mission.* Retrieved October 6, 2011, from http://www.sherpa.ac.uk/about.html

SHERPA. (2006b). *Authors and open access.* Retrieved October 6, 2011, from http://www.sherpa.ac.uk/guidance/authors.html

SHERPA. (2006c). *SHERPA services.* Retrieved October 6, 2011, from http://www.sherpa.ac.uk/index.html

University of Chicago Press. (2010). *The Chicago manual of style: The essential guide for writers, editors, and publishers* (16th ed.). Chicago: Author.

U.S. Copyright Office. (2006). *Copyright in general.* Retrieved from http://www.copyright.gov/help/faq/faq-general.html#what

U.S. Copyright Office. (2009). *Circular 92: Copyright law of the United States and related laws contained in Title 17 of the United States Code.* Retrieved October 6, 2011, from http://www.copyright.gov/title17/circ92.pdf

Veen, W., & Vrakking, B. (2006). *Homo zappiens: Growing up in a digital age.* New York: Bloomsbury.

7

Why Style Is Important

CHRISTINA A. DAVIS

A foolish consistency is the hobgoblin of little minds, adored by little statesmen and philosophers and divines.

—Ralph Waldo Emerson (n.d.)

I like consistency. If you've had a childhood like mine, you want some things you can rely on to stay the same.

—Norman Wisdom (n.d.)

Throughout their careers, writers working on their thesis or dissertation, submitting an article to a periodical, or writing a book under contract receive "instructions for authors" from their respective university or publisher. These guidelines explain preferences for manuscript page length or number of words, margins and fonts, topics to discuss, and editorial style.

AMA, AP, APA, Bluebook, Chicago, GPO, MLA, and Turabian are just a few of the shorthand notations for style that writers are likely to encounter in health care, medical, and social sciences writing (see Box 7.1). Understanding this alphabet soup, however, can be vexing. New writers, especially students, may find themselves so concerned with learning the myriad rules for imposing order on content that they concentrate more on, for example, *capitalizing words than on writing them.* Experienced writers

BOX 7.1.
EXAMPLES OF STYLE AND USAGE GUIDES

Style Guides
AMA Style
American Medical Association. (2007). *AMA manual of style: A guide for authors and editors* (10th ed.). New York: Oxford University Press. Often used in medicine. Online help is available at http://www.amamanualofstyle.com/oso/public/index.html

AP Style
Associated Press. (2012). *The Associated Press stylebook and briefing on media law* (47th ed.). New York: Basic Books. Often used in magazines and news publications. Online help is available at http://www.apstylebook.com/

APA Style
American Psychological Association. (2010). *Publication manual of the American Psychological Association* (6th ed.). Washington, DC: Author. Often used in mental health, social sciences, and education. Online help is available at http://www.apastyle.org/

Bluebook Style
Harvard Law Review Association. (2010). *The Bluebook: A uniform system of citation* (19th ed.). Cambridge, MA: Author. Often used in legal publications. Online help is available at https://www.legalbluebook.com/

Chicago (and Turabian) Style
University of Chicago Press. (2010). *The Chicago manual of style: The essential guide for writers, editors, and publishers* (16th ed.). Chicago: Author. Often used in the social and biological sciences.

may become annoyed at seemingly arcane rules of, for example, referencing, and disregard the publisher's needs. Either situation can undermine a writer's chances of completing a project or getting published.

This brief chapter is not intended to give an overview of a particular style or to argue for one's superiority over another. It does explain, from the perspective of a publishing professional, editorial style and why writers should pay attention to it.

BOX 7.1.
EXAMPLES OF STYLE AND USAGE GUIDES *(cont.)*

Chicago (and Turabian) Style (cont.)
Turabian, K. L. (2007). *A manual for writers of research papers, theses, and dissertations: Chicago style for students and researchers* (7th ed., rev. by W. C. Booth, G. G. Colomb, J. M. Williams, & University of Chicago Press Editorial Staff). Chicago: University of Chicago Press. Often used in education. Online help is available at http://www.chicagomanualofstyle.org/home.html

GPO Style
U.S. Government Printing Office. (2008). *U.S. Government Printing Office style manual* (30th ed.). Washington, DC: Author. Often used in the federal government (and by its contractors). Available online at http://www.gpo.gov/fdsys/search/pagedetails.action?granuleId=&packageId=GPO-STYLEMANUAL-2008&fromBrowse=true

MLA Style
Modern Language Association of America. (2008). *MLA style manual and guide to scholarly publishing* (3rd ed.). New York: Author. Often used in education. Online help is available at http://www.mla.org/style

Classic Guides to Usage
Strunk, W., Jr., & White, E. B. (2000). *The elements of style* (4th ed.). Needham Heights, MA: Allyn & Bacon. (Original work published 1935)
Walsh, B. (2004). *The elephants of style: A trunkload of tips on the big issues and gray areas of contemporary American English.* New York: McGraw-Hill.
Zinsser, W. (2006). *On writing well: The classic guide to writing nonfiction.* New York: HarperCollins. (Original work published 1976)

What *Style* Is

Style in this chapter refers to *usage*, not to an author's *voice*. *Style* can be defined as simply as "the rules or guidelines a publisher observes to ensure clear, consistent presentation in scholarly articles" (American Psychological Association [APA], 2010, p. 87) or in more detail as "rules related to capitalization, spelling, hyphenation, and abbreviations; punctuation, including ellipsis points, parentheses, and quotation marks; and the way numbers are treated" (University of Chicago Press, 2010, p. 70). Combined, these two views govern the way style is viewed by many publishers, including AOTA Press.

Why Style Is Important

BACKGROUND

When I was first learning the craft of editing in the late 1980s and early 1990s, my employers emphasized perfect communication. Publishing staff, who often were otherwise unemployed former English majors, fretted for hours over a document's incorrect grammar (e.g., is it "staff is" or "staff are"?), the fabrication of jargon (e.g., adding *ize* to a noun sounds important, but the result often is not a real word), misspellings (e.g., *affect* and *effect* can be confusing in mental health usage), converting U.S. measurements to metric (e.g., what exactly is a *pascal?*), and adding percentages to 100 (e.g., is it rounding or a data error?). Editors were compensated and promoted in accordance with their error rates.

Perfect sentences, statistics, paragraphs, articles, books, or journal volumes were the goal of almost every scholarly publisher. For authors, being free of mistakes in their work showed they were excellent teachers, scientists, or professionals. For publishers, consistency meant that they could attract the best authors as well as lead the marketplace in sales. Strict adherence to style made perfection easier to obtain.

Not all authors subscribed to this thinking. I sometimes spent an afternoon on the telephone explaining style points to authors who found the application of these rules contrary to teachings from a much-feared grammar school educator or university faculty advisor. When we could not convince an author that our publication's needs were appropriate, we acquiesced to that author's preferences, which, once printed alongside other articles or chapters, looked like either the author or we had made a mistake. So, while treating seriously our authors' concerns, we tried not to allow exceptions to our style rules.

Profit and favorable comparison also were factors in the selection of style, especially as some publishers had developed their editorial styles with such rigor that other publishers wanted to adopt them. The style itself was another avenue for making money. Although I have been using APA style since 1994—and was honored to have managed the editing of and develop derivative products to the 5th edition (APA, 2001)—APA has been using and later selling some version of this style since 1929 (APA, 2010). The University of Chicago has been selling its style guide, now at 1,056 pages, in earnest since 1969 and first developed the style in 1906 (University of Chicago Press, 2010). Over time, both have become predominant styles in social sciences and education writing, and using these styles informed authors and readers that a publisher was serious about its business.

NEW REALITIES

In a world of *publish ahead of print* (i.e., publishing before editing), continuous publication, and information delivery via unedited texts and 140-character "tweets," it would seem that applying an editorial style to writing is old-fashioned. In the aftermath of a global recession, fewer publishers have the staff or funding to seek perfection. These realities would seem to signal the end of style as we have known it.

Today, instead of producing error-free information, many publishers are striving to produce content that is free from *major* errors (i.e., those that would be embarrassing or legally problematic)—content that is "good enough" versus perfect—while still looking professional. Many publishers (but not all) are still relying on adherence to style to develop content that is consistent, if not always perfect.

To maximize editors' time and to allow them to concentrate more on the substance of the writing to avoid major problems, publishers have invested in affordable automated line-editing programs (e.g., eXtyles) to highlight and correct errors in a work, including style errors. Because applying an editing program might cost, for example, $30 an article, and hiring a human editor, $500 an article, having an editor correct style errors is not always a good use of a publisher's budget.

In addition, advances in technology have made the world a smaller place, and style is used to enhance understanding across cultures and

> Instead of producing error-free information, many publishers are striving to produce content that is free from *major* errors (i.e., those that would be embarrassing or legally problematic)—content that is "good enough" versus perfect—while still looking professional.

languages. For example, Unicode language from the International Organization for Standardization, featured in Chicago style, was meant to create a standard adopted worldwide for abbreviations (e.g., US instead of U.S.; University of Chicago Press, 2010), much like Latin was used as the language to name flora and fauna in the mid-1700s. Not only does this help increase the use of American-based research and knowledge around the world, but also it allows for easier translations. New readers and versions of content can bring additional revenue to publishers beleaguered by rising manufacturing costs and dwindling profit margins—and also royalties to authors (see Chapter 14).

For authors, these realities mean that not following instructions could, instead of prompting a telephone call or e-mail from a friendly editor, cause an article to be returned without consideration. In addition, authors who have a pattern of ignoring a publisher's instructions, especially if that publisher has had to repeatedly spend more than budgeted to prepare content for publication, could find themselves working with a second-tier publisher or without a publisher—even authors who are considered authorities on a particular topic.

THE CONTRARIAN VIEW

The views in this chapter are guided by my employment history in the biological and social sciences and health care, as well as by my dealings with other publishers whom I encounter in my day-to-day work. The contrarian view, for the most part arriving from non-STM (i.e., science, technology, medical) writers and publishers, is that style is unimportant in today's world of instant communication. However, for STM students, professionals, and researchers, consistency in communication will be paramount in the future, especially in the changing landscapes of science and health care. Writing and publishing in the "voice"—the language and personality—of a particular profession can give legitimacy to one's work (Stewart, 2008).

> Writing and publishing in the "voice"—the language and personality—of a particular profession can give legitimacy to one's work.

Finding Style Resources

Adhering to style is still important in today's world, and authors have a variety of ways to help navigate through the details. For example, it is common for the author of a thesis or dissertation to hire an editor to put that document into the university's preferred style so the author can concentrate instead on the content and research that inform the paper. Thesis and dissertation editors often are recommended through the university and charge by the hour, page, or job.

Also, the publishers of certain styles have created Web sites to provide guidance. For example, APA offers an "APA Style Help" page featuring online courses, blogs, and access to experts to assist authors in resolving style issues (APA, 2012). Chicago has an online site that allows writers and editors to create their own manual, highlighting style points used most often and personalizing their own style sheets (University of Chicago Press, 2012).

During the past few decades, the number of publisher exceptions to the application of style has grown, as content has become more personalized to readers. Even the arbiters of style recognize this: "The *Publication Manual* presents explicit style requirements but acknowledges that alternatives are sometimes necessary; authors should balance the rules of the *Publication Manual* with good judgment" (APA, 1994, p. xxiii). Although APA is the foundation for AOTA's editorial style, AOTA Press staff use a 94-page guide of clarifications and exceptions to it (AOTA, 2012), because the lexicon of occupational therapy is different from that of psychology. Further, different product lines from the same publisher can have different styles (e.g., legal works follow Bluebook, everything else follows APA). Many publishers (and universities) post their author guidelines and exceptions on their Web sites or include them with contracts and other paperwork.

Applying the Style

Like all types of style, editorial style is always adapting to changing realities and tastes. Using resources to appropriately apply a publisher's style—thus, following *all* of a publisher's instructions—can help authors publish more successfully. Paying attention to style requirements shows a publisher that an author is serious about the project. A publisher then is likely to invest more time and funding in that author, and the work produced from that partnership will look professional and consistent with other important works in the field.

> **Like all types of style, editorial style is always adapting to changing realities and tastes.**

REFERENCES

American Medical Association. (2007). *AMA manual of style: A guide for authors and editors* (10th ed.). New York: Oxford University Press.

American Occupational Therapy Association. (2012, October). *AOTA Press style guide*. Bethesda, MD: AOTA Press.

American Psychological Association. (1929). Instructions in regard to preparation of manuscript. *Psychological Bulletin, 26,* 57–63.

American Psychological Association. (1994). *Publication manual of the American Psychological Association* (4th ed.). Washington, DC: Author.

American Psychological Association. (2001). *Publication manual of the American Psychological Association* (5th ed.). Washington, DC: Author.

American Psychological Association. (2010). *Publication manual of the American Psychological Association* (6th ed.). Washington, DC: Author.

American Psychological Association. (2012). *APA style help*. Available online at http://www.apastyle.org/apa-style-help.aspx

Associated Press. (2012). *The Associated Press stylebook and briefing on media law* (47th ed.). New York: Basic Books.

Emerson, R. W. (n.d.). Consistency. Available online at http://www.brainyquote.com/quotes/keywords/consistency.html#oYwIFrT2QXsx8ISF.99

Harvard Law Review Association. (2010). *The Bluebook: A uniform system of citation* (19th ed.). Cambridge, MA: Author.

Modern Language Association of America. (2008). *MLA style manual and guide to scholarly publishing* (3rd ed.). New York: Author.

Stewart, S. (2008). *Style is strategy: How editorial standards send your message.* San Francisco: Thinkshift. Available online at http://thinkshiftcom.com/articles/TS_article_style.pdf

Strunk, W., Jr., & White, E. B. (2000). *The elements of style* (4th ed.). Needham Heights, MA: Allyn & Bacon. (Original work published 1935)

Turabian, K. L. (2007). *A manual for writers of research papers, theses, and dissertations: Chicago style for students and researchers* (7th ed., rev. by W. C. Booth, G. G. Colomb, J. M. Williams, & University of Chicago Press Editorial Staff). Chicago: University of Chicago Press.

University of Chicago Press. (1969). *The Chicago manual of style* (12th ed.). Chicago: Author.

University of Chicago Press. (2010). *The Chicago manual of style: The essential guide for writers, editors, and publishers* (16th ed.). Chicago: Author.

University of Chicago Press. (2012). *The Chicago Manual of Style online.* Available online at http://www.chicagomanualofstyle.org/home.html

U.S. Government Printing Office. (2008). *U.S. Government Printing Office style manual* (30th ed.). Washington, DC: Author.

Walsh, B. (2004). *The elephants of style: A trunkload of tips on the big issues and gray areas of contemporary American English.* New York: McGraw-Hill.

Wisdom, N. (n.d.). Consistency. Available online at http://www.brainyquote.com /quotes/keywords/consistency.html#oYwIFrT2QXsx8ISF.99

Zinsser, W. (2006). *On writing well: The classic guide to writing nonfiction.* New York: HarperCollins. (Original work published 1976.)

Writing for Your Audience

8

The Heart of the Struggle: Using Project Management to Overcome Obstacles to Writing a Dissertation

ALISON B. MILLER, PhD

Writing is like driving at night in the fog. You can only see as far as your headlights, but you can make the whole trip that way.

—E. L. Doctorow (1988)

I t's late at night. You find yourself sitting at your computer with the intention of making progress on your thesis or dissertation writing project. Yet you are procrastinating or working ineffectively. You keep checking your e-mail, surfing the Internet, playing computer games, rewriting sentences obsessively, or doing more "research" even though there are piles of articles on your desk and the floor around you. The next day, you wake up anxious at the time that is passing without your having completed any meaningful writing.

Quickly, you think of a solution. You imagine yourself producing high-quality writing in a short amount of time, and you devise a to-do list that helps you feel better and more in control. But this improvement in your mood is short-lived because, in truth, this list is merely an anxiety management tool, not an honest reflection of your own writing process or of what you can realistically do on a day-to-day basis. One or two days later, you feel demoralized again and discouraged that you can't stick to a plan.

Writing is hard. Writing a thesis, dissertation, or scholarly paper is uniquely hard. High-stakes scholarly writing challenges you to think critically and conceptually as you stretch your intellectual abilities and your personality to write a sound paper and meet the demands and expectations of the faculty or editors who are the gatekeepers to your success. Writing involves substantial effort and struggle, even for experienced writers. Anyone who writes with ease has spent years writing, integrating feedback from others and developing their skills as a writer.

Many believe that other writers write with little effort and angst. But writing is rarely as easy as it may seem to external observers. People tend to compare their internal experience of life to what they see externally in others. From that point of view, they often see themselves as inadequate in comparison. But you can't really know what writing is like on the inside for others. Perhaps other writers are getting more help from their advisor or mentor or are working with a writing coach. And even if it really is easier for some, it doesn't mean that you can't get better at writing with practice, persistence, and the help of others.

In reality, writing is a challenge for most people and even for most other writers. The good news is that you can learn new and better ways to approach writing.

In this chapter, I describe skills, strategies, and an approach to writing that can help you increase your effectiveness and productivity as a writer. For more than 12 years, I have been a dissertation coach, helping thousands of graduate students, both in workshops and groups and individually, to successfully overcome writing challenges and complete their doctoral dissertations and master's theses. This chapter is not a technical manual or how-to guide about the components of sound dissertation and thesis writing; rather, it is a guide to overcoming common psychological obstacles that make writing a challenge, developing a positive writing mindset, and using a structured approach to writing.

If you feel challenged, overwhelmed, scared, or just plain inadequate, I can promise you are not alone. Learning a new approach to writing is possible, no matter how much you have struggled in the past. Although the chapter is aimed specifically at graduate students, anyone who struggles to write can use the ideas in this chapter to successfully complete their writing projects.

Overcoming Procrastination and Perfectionism

Procrastination and perfectionism are behavioral patterns that interfere with the ability to write consistently and productively.

Procrastination and perfectionism are behavioral patterns that interfere with the ability to write consistently and productively. It is common for writers to experience one or the other or even both. In this section I offer an understanding of what fuels procrastination and perfectionism and how you can break free from these patterns and change your behavior for the better.

PROCRASTINATION

Procrastination is a form of avoidance and includes anything you do—from the obvious (e.g., checking e-mail, spending hours on social networking Web sites, watching TV) to the less obvious (e.g., conducting another literature search instead of reading the articles you already have)—that involves actively delaying or avoiding your dissertation or thesis work. Engaging in any of these activities is not necessarily bad. In fact, meaningful breaks from your work help you rejuvenate and make better use of your writing time. It is a problem only when you engage in such activities to the exclusion of doing meaningful work. You are bound to procrastinate, but you can learn to procrastinate less. The first step to changing your ways is to understand what is really going on when you procrastinate.

It is easy to believe that you are lazy when you are procrastinating. Yet laziness implies apathy about taking action, whereas procrastination is a process of actively avoiding taking action that you are committed to doing (Knaus, 2002). Sure, there may be times when you feel apathetic toward your project, but rather than being genuinely apathetic, it is more likely that you are feeling uncomfortable in some way and would like to avoid those uncomfortable thoughts and feelings. The easiest way to avoid your thoughts and feelings is to avoid your dissertation or thesis. Thus, when you are procrastinating, it is not your work that you are avoiding; it is your thoughts and feelings about your work that you are avoiding. To reduce how much you procrastinate, begin by increasing your awareness of what you are thinking and feeling in relation to your dissertation and thesis writing.

Many people who write experience negative thoughts about themselves and the writing experience. They often have self-defeating thoughts about their own skills, abilities, and intelligence (e.g., "The faculty made a mistake letting me in this program." "I'm not smart enough." "I'm not smart; I just work hard and know how to fool people into thinking I am intelligent." "I don't really have what it takes to finish my dissertation."; Miller, 2009). Frequent thoughts about failure create a great deal of fear (e.g., "What if I write an entire dissertation and fail my defense?" "What if no one will hire me after I finish?" "I'm scared my advisor will rip my dissertation to shreds and tell me to start over."). These negative thoughts tell you that you or your writing is inadequate in some important way, make high demands for the quality and quantity of writing, and insist that you meet these demands or risk looking unintelligent or inadequate.

Thoughts such as these are unpleasant to experience, and understandably a person thinking these thoughts would rather move away from them. These thoughts also have very real emotional consequences. When your mind is telling you that you are inadequate or making unrealistic demands for your performance, it is likely you will feel anxious, fearful, stressed, and possibly even ashamed or depressed. It is also common for writers to feel guilty, angry, frustrated, and demoralized when they are not progressing on their project as they believe they should be.

Human beings naturally seek to avoid pain and to control and stop anything that creates pain or discomfort (Hayes, Strosahl, & Wilson, 1999). Procrastination is actually a specific manifestation of a behavior called *experiential avoidance*, which is any behavior that helps you avoid or escape unwanted and unpleasant thoughts and feelings (as well as unpleasant body sensations, such as heart racing or chest tightness; Hayes et al., 1999). Behaviors such as the common procrastination behaviors mentioned earlier are all forms of experiential avoidance if the intention of the behavior is to avoid or escape unwanted thoughts and feelings about your dissertation or thesis (Miller, 2009).

The next time you catch yourself putting off writing or struggling to stay engaged once you are writing, tune in to yourself and what you are experiencing. What are you thinking? What are you feeling? What are you experiencing that you find unpleasant and would like to avoid? You may want to write down your answers on paper so you can obtain some distance from your thoughts and feelings and more clearly see what it is that you are avoiding.

For example, as I wrote the first draft of this section, I felt very uncertain about how to organize my writing and what key points I wanted to express. I also had some concerns about what the people at the American Occupational Therapy Association (AOTA) who asked me to write this chapter would think of my writing and the content of the chapter. I worried that this chapter would not meet their expectations and that the person from AOTA who personally invited me to write this chapter would be embarrassed that she had extended the opportunity to me. One afternoon, when I intended to write a rough initial draft of this very section, I kept playing solitaire, checking my e-mail, and making tea.

Ironic, isn't it? There I was writing about procrastination and engaging in it simultaneously! What was going on with me? I was avoiding my self-doubting thoughts, concerns, and anxiety about my ability to perform. Even a dissertation coach can get caught in avoidance mode. Fortunately, I followed my own advice and jotted down on paper my fears and concerns. Doing so gave me the freedom to refocus on writing and write a really rough draft, even with those fears and concerns in the background.

PERFECTIONISM

Like procrastination, perfectionism is a form of avoidance. *Perfectionism* is the belief that standards lower than perfection are unacceptable (Hewitt & Flett, 1991). For example, you have perfectionistic tendencies if you obsess over word choice or the phrasing of sentences in an effort to get it perfect. Perfectionists are usually concerned about looking intellectually inadequate and fear negative consequences from failing to meet their own or others' extremely high expectations of them.

How does perfectionism lead to avoidance? The aim of perfectionistic behavior is to avoid the unpleasant thoughts (e.g., "I am not smart enough" or "I'll never get a job if I don't write a stellar dissertation") and feelings (e.g., worthlessness, anxiety, inadequacy) you anticipate will arise when your work is criticized or of a quality you deem unacceptable. There is nothing wrong with having high standards for the end product of your writing project. But standards that are too high early in the writing process fuel procrastination and paralyze your attempts at meaningful progress.

Perfectionism also severely curbs your freedom as a writer. Instead of fostering experimentation, exploration, and creativity, which allow you to fully and meaningfully engage in the writing experience, the drive for perfection dictates rules and absolute standards you must achieve. It prevents you from being flexible, open, and innovative as you express ideas in words. Perfectionism often has a strong grip on those who experience it, and it can take time to release perfectionistic tendencies. So be patient and, more important, be compassionate with yourself. Being perfectionistic is hard enough without judging yourself for being this way.

As with procrastination, it is important to increase your awareness of the perfectionistic thoughts and feelings you are avoiding if you want to break free. Increased awareness sets the stage for you to develop a more accepting stance toward the thoughts and feelings you avoid. Such acceptance then creates an opportunity to take action aligned with your values and goals instead of being stuck in avoidance. The section that follows takes a closer look at ways to develop an accepting stance toward troublesome thoughts and feelings and take action aligned with your values.

LOOSENING THE GRIP OF PROCRASTINATION AND PERFECTIONISM: ACCEPTANCE AND VALUE-DRIVEN ACTION

No magic spell will easily and quickly resolve patterns of procrastination and perfectionism. However, there is an effective way to reduce these behaviors and increase your freedom to write effectively and efficiently. As a dissertation coach, I use an approach to reduce procrastination and perfectionism based in a psychotherapy called *Acceptance and Commitment Therapy* developed by Steven Hayes and his colleagues (Hayes & Smith, 2005; Hayes et al., 1999). This approach is fundamentally about accepting yourself, others, and your thoughts and feelings with compassion; choosing valued directions and goals for your life; and committing to taking action aligned with your values and value-driven goals (Eifert & Forsyth, 2005; Hayes et al., 1999).

Learning to accept thoughts and feelings that fuel procrastination and perfectionism is vital to loosening the grip of these behavior patterns. First, it is necessary to understand what is meant by *acceptance*. In Acceptance and Commitment Therapy, acceptance is about being willing to experience unpleasant or unwanted thoughts and feelings in the service of taking action aligned with your values and value-driven goals (Eifert & Forsyth, 2005). It is not passive acceptance, in which you give up taking action or tolerate or condone your private experience. Instead, it is an active form of acceptance in which you witness the thoughts and feelings that you are having and acknowledge their presence without demanding that they not be there.

Such willingness grants you the freedom to be in the moment with unwanted cognitive and emotional experiences instead of reacting to them with behavior (e.g., procrastination, perfectionism) that is designed to avoid these experiences (Hayes et al., 1999; Miller, 2009). Certainly you can seek to directly change your thoughts and feelings to be more positive. At times you may be successful. However, research shows that changing and controlling thoughts and feelings is not easy. In fact, the more you try to change or suppress thoughts and feelings you don't like, the more they tend to stick around and even become amplified (Hayes et al., 1999). Because it is very difficult to control or suppress unwanted thoughts and feelings, acceptance is a better antidote.

When you learn that you can accept and be with any thoughts or feelings that arise within you, you come to see that thoughts and feelings are something you have. Your thoughts and feelings no longer have you in their grip, dictating how you behave. You can then better direct your energy and behavior in the directions that matter most to you.

For example, if you are experiencing anxiety and negative thoughts about your intelligence, acceptance is about being willing to allow those experiences to exist within you without reacting to them through avoidance. Through acceptance, you begin to consider that you can have self-doubting thoughts and anxiety at the same time that you write. You can see that the thought "I am not smart enough" is merely an evaluation your mind makes in connection to writing your literature review and that anxiety is a feeling you feel.

Thoughts and feelings are not true or false. They simply are experiences human beings have. By looking at them this way, you can better see that you have the freedom to act as you choose. Unwanted thoughts and feelings and writing are no longer mutually exclusive. You are able to free up the energy you have been spending trying to control and suppress negative thoughts and feelings to actually work on your dissertation or thesis.

Being aware of what you value and why completing your dissertation or thesis is important to you will help you take action when you would normally avoid your thoughts and feelings. In the midst of all of your roles and responsibilities and the pressure to finish graduate school, you may lose sight of your values and purpose in life.

Values are the intangible qualities you believe are important to demonstrate in your life. Unlike your goals in life, which are ways for you to live out and express your values, your values are not something you can achieve: They provide ongoing direction to your life, guiding the choices you make on a day-to-day basis.

When you consider your choice to earn a graduate degree and pursue an education in occupational therapy, for example, consider the values that guided this choice. Do you value making a difference or contribution, creativity, collaboration, learning, growth, or accomplishment? Spend some time considering what really matters to you in your life and the legacy you want to leave as a human being. What do you want to be known for? What impact do you want to have on others? What qualities do you want to demonstrate in your life? Such an inquiry can help you be more aware of your most important values. Consider engaging in this inquiry over time and recording your values in writing.

When it comes to breaking free from procrastination and perfectionism, awareness of what you value matters. Knowing what you value gives you a sense of the direction to move in, even when you experience thoughts and feelings you would rather avoid. In this way, you commit yourself to take action that is aligned with your values and your value-driven goals and to allow unpleasant, unwanted thoughts and feelings to be in your experience at the same time. So how do you move forward toward your values when you are experiencing negative thoughts and feelings?

I find a bus metaphor to be very useful to understand and apply this idea of taking action aligned with your values in the presence of unwanted or unpleasant thoughts and feelings. Imagine being on a city bus. When you are on a bus, there is a bus driver and there are passengers. The bus driver drives the bus down the street headed in a particular direction—let's say, headed toward 95th Street. She drives down the street and stops regularly so passengers can get on and off. The bus driver does not determine who gets on and off the bus or when they do so.

Most of the passengers who get on the bus are pleasant or neutral. They pay the fare, have a seat, ride the bus until they reach their destination, and exit the bus. But at times, unpleasant, undesirable passengers get on the bus. These passengers may talk loudly on their cell phones, solicit other passengers, argue with the bus driver, or be distracting or disruptive in some other way. Now if the bus driver wants to keep driving in the direction of 95th Street, she has to accept that some of the passengers on her bus are unwanted and unpleasant. If she is not willing to carry those passengers on the bus, then she must stop the bus, get out of her seat, and try to get the passengers off the bus. She becomes involved in a struggle to get rid of unwanted passengers and consequently is no longer able to drive the bus in the direction of 95th Street.

As a writer, you are the bus driver with a specific destination: living by your values and successfully earning a graduate degree. As you write your dissertation or thesis, all kinds of "passengers" will get on your bus in the form of thoughts, feelings, or even the urge to watch television or head to the fridge. And they *will* get on the bus, whether you want them to or not. Many of those passengers cooperate with writing effectively. Yet it is also common to have passengers who do not. Thoughts such as "I am not smart enough" or "My dissertation needs to be perfect" or emotions such as anxiety or boredom can board your bus at any time.

When you get caught up in procrastination or perfectionism, you have basically stopped driving in the direction of your values and value-driven goals. You may be waiting for your unwanted passengers to get off the bus or trying to get control of them so you can get back to writing. Maybe you are not even aware that they are on the bus; you just know that you don't feel like writing or that you have stopped writing effectively. When procrastination and perfectionism take hold of you, more passengers may get on the bus, such as "You're lazy" or "What's wrong with you? Why can't you just sit down and write?" or "You should get your act together," as well as guilt, panic, and feelings of being overwhelmed. This second round of passengers can fuel even more procrastination and perfectionism and make it even harder to drive the bus.

So how can you drive in the direction of finishing your writing project with a busload of unwanted thoughts and feelings? The first step is to acknowledge that you are, in fact, caught in procrastination or perfectionism and then to observe what thoughts and feelings are present. Acknowledge these passengers. Allow yourself to fully witness their existence, and grant them permission to be on the bus. If you can release the demand that unwanted thoughts and feelings not be present for you to be able to write and instead develop a more accepting stance toward them, they will have far less power to shape your behavior. When you are willing to let unwanted passengers be on the bus and can hold space for them and be present with them without judgment, you give yourself much greater freedom to take action aligned with your values and commitments.

I encourage you to keep welcoming unwanted passengers on your bus. Let them know they are free to have a seat and that you will be driving and writing your project one step at a time, no matter how rowdy and challenging they may be.

Embrace the Process of Writing

Another important way to overcome obstacles to writing is to learn to embrace the process and experience of writing. People often believe they should be able to just sit down and write something of good quality without a lot of effort. I think of this as a product-oriented approach to writing. If you have developed this approach, you likely write with the intention of bypassing rough drafts or anything that you would not want others to read. You sit down to write and aim to create the end product, or at least a high-quality draft. You don't want to feel stuck or stupid or write rough sentences or paragraphs that you know you will need to revise later—you want to get it done. Now, you may not consciously think about it quite that way. Rationally, you understand that writing is hard and takes a lot of effort. But such rational thought often flies out the window when writing does not come easily or takes longer than you think it should.

It is critical for people to come to terms with a basic reality: Writing is a process, a practiced activity that evolves over time and requires, by design, effort, persistence, creativity, and revision. Academic and professional writing is full of false starts, errors, awkward phrasing, organizational challenges, lack of clarity, and difficulty adequately or accurately describing concepts, theory, research design, analytic techniques, or implications of the findings and limitations of the research. Sure, there are times when writing flows and you are "in the zone," churning out one great sentence after another. It is great when that happens. But such episodes are often fleeting, and it is not long before you end up in the land where writing is an ambiguous, confusing, and even scary process. But don't despair. There is a way to work through this reality of the writing experience: The way to get through is to learn to embrace the process.

> Academic and professional writing is full of false starts, errors, awkward phrasing, organizational challenges, lack of clarity, and difficulty adequately or accurately describing concepts, theory, research design, analytic techniques, or implications of the findings and limitations of the research.

What do I mean by "embrace the process"? I encourage you to develop a process-oriented approach to writing in which you discover your own method of writing and let go of the mythological version in which writing occurs naturally without a lot of effort, struggle, rough drafts, or feedback from others. By seeking to develop a process-oriented approach to writing, you will likely be a more effective and productive writer in the long run.

FOCUS ON PROCESS VS. PRODUCT

The *process* of writing a dissertation or thesis involves many steps and may include activities such as research, reading, taking notes, outlining, drafting, revising (often many times), and incorporating the feedback of others. At the end of that process, the *product* of your efforts is created. The difference between process and product seems obvious on paper, yet in the practice of writing they are often confused.

One of the main reasons we confuse the process of writing with the product of writing is that we rarely have the opportunity to view how writing actually occurs for other people. When you read someone else's dissertation, a published journal article, or a book, you see only the end product and rarely, if ever, all the false starts, rough drafts, feedback from editors and reviewers, and revisions. Nor do other writers generally share their rough drafts or writing difficulties with much candor. So you don't get many opportunities to view the evolution of writing in the process of becoming a product.

A few years ago, I wrote a book, *Finish Your Dissertation Once and for All* (Miller, 2009), and the experience of writing the book taught me a lot about having a process-oriented versus product-oriented approach to writing. For the first 6 months after I received the book contract from the publisher, I wrote nothing. And I mean absolutely nothing at all. Once again, you can laugh at the irony, given that my book is largely about overcoming psychological obstacles to doing a dissertation (including procrastination) and being an effective writer. Even once I got started, I wrote haphazardly for several months, never fully committing to writing. Eventually I got it together and wrote the book. I even ended up enjoying the process, especially revising the book after I received feedback from my editor.

What happened? Why did I wait so long to get started? And how did I eventually get going? Even though I had made it through the process of writing a master's thesis and dissertation, the prospect of writing a book seemed daunting, and I got caught up in avoidance mode. I was required to go through peer review once I wrote the book, and because of my prior experiences with that process, I feared snarky comments, harsh criticism, and the possibility that I would fail to produce a text my publisher would find worthy of publication. Also, I knew my book would end up on Amazon.com and other Web sites where people could write whatever they liked in a review.

There were, of course, other distractions in my life: I had a baby, a 5-year-old daughter, and a busy coaching practice, so carving out time to write was a challenge. But my own fears posed the biggest problem. I was essentially in a holding pattern in which I contemplated getting started while I waited for more time and confidence to magically appear. In the meantime, I made lots of work plans but not much progress.

During lunch with a good friend who had written a book, I recognized how I was not practicing what I preach. I realize this seems very obvious, but somehow in the months I was putting off writing, I had turned a blind eye to reality. I had lost sight of the difference between the process of writing a book and the end product that is created in the process. I was so focused on the product and whether it would be adequate and meet expectations that I was forgetting to engage in the process—that is, the actual writing. The part of me that worries "I'm not smart or adequate enough" wanted to skip the process and create a high-quality product without a lot of effort. Of course, that is an entirely unattainable goal that only served to paralyze me. The desire to skip the process is a seductive trap for anyone engaged in writing.

When I recommitted to the process of writing and let myself just write without considering what others would think, I had a breakthrough. I opened myself up to the idea that there are likely many ways I could approach writing the book and that I would use this experience as an opportunity to discover and even create my own writing process. Letting go of the desire to bypass the process (which I let go of over and over again) helped me develop a fruitful process for my own writing.

Here is how it went for me:

1. I created an outline of the key points I wanted to make in each chapter (these points evolved and developed as I wrote the chapter).
2. I refined the list of points and ended up with what looked like a detailed informal outline.
3. I wrote a really rough draft longhand, one point at a time.
4. I typed up my handwritten work, editing frequently as I typed.
5. I printed the typed writing and edited it on paper.
6. I entered the editing, printed the revised version, and edited it again on paper.

I repeated Steps 5 and 6 many times. Sure, there were times when I got stuck and began avoiding my writing, but overall, I was better able to write page after page.

A good deal of the initial writing I did was never seen by anyone else and required a lot of editing (both by myself and by others). But I was engaged in writing, and it was the writing I needed to do to get me to the writing that would eventually become the product on the bookshelf.

In truth, no written product exists without a writing process. No dissertation, thesis, research article, or book has ever been written without a process to create it over time. Even if you are already quite comfortable with the process of writing, we all get stuck, and when you find yourself fixated on the product, try a process-oriented approach to writing. Three strategies useful in this approach are cultivating a growth mindset, writing really rough drafts, and asking for help.

CULTIVATE A GROWTH MINDSET

One of the most important ways to fully embrace a process-oriented approach is to cultivate what is known as a *growth mindset*. Carol Dweck (2002, 2006), a psychologist and researcher, identified two key mindsets, or sets of beliefs, that people have about intelligence. These two mindsets have a profound impact on people's response to challenges and failures, their motivation, and ultimately their actual performance and capacity to strengthen their intellect, skills, and abilities (Dweck, 2002, 2006). The mindsets are called the *fixed mindset* and the *growth mindset,* and each involves several key beliefs.

People who have a fixed mindset believe that intelligence is fixed or unchangeable and that they have a finite amount. Because they don't know at what level their intelligence is fixed, they use their performance on intellectual or academic tasks to evaluate how intelligent they are (Dweck, 2002). If they perform well, they deem themselves intelligent. If they perform poorly, they fear they are not smart.

Generally, people with a fixed mindset exert a lot of effort making sure they look smart and believe they must avoid looking unintelligent. In addition, they believe that their current performance is indicative of their long-term potential (e.g., how smart I am now and how well I perform now are how I will always be) and that if they were truly intelligent, they would not need to put in a lot of effort to achieve highly (Dweck, 2002). These people believe not only that their performance measures intelligence, but also that it measures self-worth. Thus, poor performance often contributes to feelings of worthlessness.

In response to being challenged intellectually, students with a fixed mindset actually lower their effort for fear that they are not smart enough to meet intellectual challenges. By doing so, they can blame poor results on their effort rather than on their intelligence (Dweck, 2000). They may also engage in other self-handicapping behaviors (Dweck, 2006) such as putting off work until the last minute or failing to create opportunities to learn by soliciting feedback from others or attending a research methods or writing class. Such behavior helps them avoid being in a situation in which they may look unintelligent (e.g., not knowing how to do something, receiving critical feedback) and thus feel worthless. The bottom line is that these students don't like to struggle or put in the sustained effort it takes to succeed at writing. Thus, students with a fixed mindset can actually stunt their own intellectual growth (Dweck, 2002).

In contrast to the fixed mindset, people with a growth mindset view intelligence as malleable, as something that can be grown and developed. They believe that with effort, engagement, and persistence, they can become smarter and more capable (Dweck, 2006). Students with a growth mindset also believe that their current performance simply tells them where they are currently and what they need to do to grow intellectually. These students thrive and become more motivated to learn when they experience intellectual challenges. They are not concerned with proving they are smart enough, largely because they don't look to their performance to evaluate their intelligence, nor do they correlate intelligence or performance with their self-worth (Dweck, 2002).

Thus, their self-worth is not on the line at every turn, and they are free to learn instead of being driven to perform well as a means to preserve their sense of self-worth. They have room to write rough drafts, make mistakes, seek the input of others, and explore ideas without having to get it "right" or produce quality writing at all times. Consequently, they are better able to improve their writing over time.

Whereas students with a fixed mindset are concerned primarily with performance and looking smart, students with a growth mindset are concerned with learning. They feel smart by exerting effort, engaging with challenging tasks, and trying to solve problems. This focus on learning and investment of time and effort result in an important outcome: Students with a growth mindset perform better academically than those with a fixed mindset (Dweck, 2000). So in the end, you will write more effectively if you focus on writing as an opportunity to learn and expand your skills rather than as a performance-based test of how smart and capable you are. A growth mindset is more conducive to a process-oriented approach to writing and ultimately to a successful and satisfying writing and learning experience.

Those who have more of a fixed mindset about writing can cultivate a growth mindset. American society and our education system foster the fixed mindset by emphasizing and rewarding performance and natural talent largely to the exclusion of effort, persistence, practice, and what it really takes to learn (Dweck, 2002, 2006). Many of us in the academic world have spent a great deal of energy proving our intelligence and our worth. Recognizing these tendencies is the first meaningful step away from the fixed mindset trap.

Recognize that your beliefs about intelligence are holding you back from learning, and remember that you were not born with a fixed mindset. Babies and very young children relentlessly seek to learn and make sense of the world around them. They are curious and willing to explore and play, and they don't expect themselves to be skilled when they are learning. If they need help, they ask for it. If they try something and don't succeed, they try again. Allow yourself to reconnect with the child you once were who was not afraid to make mistakes and who didn't even see mistakes or struggle as a problem. Experience is just as much a learning process. I encourage you to continually recommit to learning instead of performing and proving yourself. You may find you need time and persistence, but that is what the growth mindset is all about.

WRITE REALLY ROUGH DRAFTS

Many writers espouse the strategy of writing very rough drafts without consideration of audience, grammar, spelling, flow, organization, sentence structure, or, most important, what anyone else will think. A really rough first draft helps you focus on the basics of what you are trying to say, even if the writing is very disorganized and unclear. This kind of drafting is about getting something down on paper so that you have something to clean up and revise and eventually turn into writing you would consider letting someone else read (Bolker, 1998; Lamott, 1994).

If you are not used to writing this way, it can feel very uncomfortable or even frightening to allow yourself to let go of high standards and just write a crappy draft. I realize it is not possible to completely let go of a focus on writing well or on what your advisor and committee will think. But it is possible to get better at writing with lower standards. And relax; you can raise your standards later before you let anyone else read your work.

Consider my volume dial technique. Imagine that you have a volume dial in front of you that goes from 1 to 10 but represents the standards for quality of your writing instead of the volume of sound. At 1, you have extremely low standards, so stream-of-consciousness writing is acceptable. At 10, you expect your writing to be polished and ready to be defended before your dissertation or thesis committee or published in a leading journal. People don't usually realize they have a choice about where they set the volume dial when they write. And many students write as if 8, 9, and 10 are the only acceptable or available options for writing. It feels safer to write with higher standards because it gives you the illusion that you can avoid the critique of others or the frustration of having to revise and rework your writing.

People often raise the volume on their standards for quality and quantity of writing as a way to jump-start productivity, especially after a period of procrastination. However, this approach often backfires; if the volume is too high, the standards are unachievable. Thus, the very strategy students devise to increase productivity creates anxiety and the feeling of being overwhelmed, leading to even more procrastination and lowered productivity (Miller, 2009). If you tend to write on high volume, be honest with yourself. Is writing this way effective? Is it really working for you? If you are not pleased with your writing progress, you procrastinate a lot, or you generally disdain the writing experience, it is likely you would benefit by turning down the volume on your standards and expectations. I have seen this approach work for many students.

Start by picking a narrow writing focus (e.g., a small subsection of your literature review, the measures section of your method) and then imagine yourself turning the volume down. You are letting go and choosing to trust that if you write with lower standards, you will later be able to turn up the volume and create a successful product. If you have little idea how to approach the section, turn down the volume to 1 or 2 and just let yourself put some ideas down on paper without worrying about writing complete sentences. I often encourage students at this point to focus on identifying the key points they want to make without worrying about getting them right. Just do your best, and if you stay engaged and persist, you will be able to articulate the key points over time. Once you are clearer on the points you want to make, you can turn up the volume a little and start writing sentences and paragraphs.

You may be thinking that this approach to writing is inefficient or takes a long time. In practice, however, students find that writing moves more quickly when they stop obsessing over sentences, using the thesaurus, and engaging in other writing behaviors that slow down the writing flow. They become much more efficient at drafting because they don't lose momentum or sight of the big picture of what they are trying to convey. They also start to realize that often the only way to figure out what they want to write is by writing. Many writers find that they really only know what they are writing once they have written it (Lamott, 1994). Dialing down your first draft to a 1, 2, or 3 can be a way to free you from the bonds of high standards, procrastination, perfectionism, and writer's block and enable you to more fully embrace a process-oriented approach.

ASK FOR HELP

Another key way to embrace a process-oriented approach to writing is to ask for help. Inevitably when you write your dissertation or thesis, you will get stuck and not know what to write or how to write it. Many students believe that they should be able to figure things out by themselves and that asking for help is a sign of weakness or lack of intelligence. Sure, writing requires independence, but that does not mean you need to write without the input of others. The truth is that all the books or journal articles you read, even if they have only one author, were influenced by the feedback, input, and editing of other people. Whenever I read a book, I always make a point of reading the author's acknowledgment of all the people who assisted him or her in creating the book. Doing so reminds me that it takes a community to produce a book even though only one person's or a few people's names end up on the cover.

When you write, you can struggle alone, or you can ask for help. I don't mean to imply that you are not capable of solving writing dilemmas

> **The truth is that all the books or journal articles you read, even if they have only one author, were influenced by the feedback, input, and editing of other people.**

and challenges on your own. I just don't believe you always need to labor alone, struggling and stymied when you could ask for help.

The mere act of talking with others can help you generate new ideas, look at your research and writing from a different angle, and discover a solution that was not previously evident. Choose someone you feel comfortable talking to about your writing and who is best suited to your particular writing issues. If your advisor tells you that you need to submit a complete draft before he or she will discuss your work, find someone who is more willing to discuss it before then. Consider forming or joining a group in which writers discuss their work, and solicit the input and feedback of other group members (Miller, 2009).

Relying heavily on your own thoughts to develop your ideas and writing is a sound approach, yet it is ultimately limiting when it is the only approach in your repertoire. Most people process information not only by thinking and writing but also by talking. You will likely find that when you talk out loud about your ideas, you are able to think, make connections, find solutions, and identify how you want to express yourself in writing. Thus, talking to others, even if they only listen to you, can be a part of your writing process and help you move through writing blocks and challenges.

There are times when you will need substantive help. You may be struggling to develop a dissertation or thesis topic. You may require help understanding how to apply a theoretical framework to your research, design your study, or develop a sound data analysis plan. On such occasions, asking for help from someone who is both knowledgeable and approachable is wise. Don't struggle alone; it will only slow you down and make conducting your dissertation an unsavory experience. And more important, you won't learn. Remember, the real purpose of being a graduate student is not only to earn a degree (the product) but also to engage meaningfully in the process so you can learn and increase your skills, knowledge, and capacity for critical thinking (the prize from the process). The higher purpose of graduate school is to grow as a human being, not to prove how smart you are.

The Project Management Approach

One of the most important elements of my dissertation coaching approach is teaching my clients to use a project management approach to dissertation and thesis (or any) writing. A project management approach is essentially breaking down the Mount Everest of writing into more manageable hills (Miller, 2009). Most of us already know that breaking down large tasks into smaller tasks is a good way to increase productivity and reduce procrastination, but I find in general that this practice is not intuitive or explicitly taught in school. So let's take a closer look at the project management approach, its benefits, and how you can use it. (For a more extensive discussion of this topic, see Miller, 2009.)

The most essential part of the project management approach I teach is using daily action plans to structure and plan what dissertation or thesis work you will do on a day-to-day basis. This approach is particularly useful for planning writing. I find that many students approach writing with plans such as "Write literature review" or "Draft Chapter 3" or, even worse, "Write dissertation," goals that are too big and ambiguous.

Table 8.1 is a basic action plan for writing. This plan is for a student seeking to write the first four sections of his methods chapter for his

TABLE 8.1. Basic 1-Week Action Plan

Date	Action
Monday	Write first draft of Setting section.
Tuesday	Write first draft of Participants section.
Wednesday	Write first draft of Measures section. Write first draft of Procedures section.
Thursday	Revise first draft of Setting section. Revise first draft of Participants section.
Friday	Revise first draft of Measures section. Revise first draft of Procedures section.
Saturday	Revise and edit second draft of Setting section. Revise and edit second draft of Participants section. Revise and edit second draft of Measures section. Revise and edit second draft of Procedures section. Write a cover note to advisor noting any questions I have about my methodology. Submit cover note and methods to my advisor for review.
Sunday	Take day off.

dissertation proposal. The pace of this plan was appropriate for him because he already had a solid outline of his method and an understanding of the setting where he would collect data, the potential study participants, his recruitment methods, and the study measures. The pace at which you work may be different depending on your other life roles and responsibilities, the length of your writing project, and how prepared you are to write a particular portion of your dissertation.

In this example of an action plan, the student broke down writing the first draft of his methods chapter into individual sections. He planned separate times for drafting and revising each of these sections before submitting the methods section to his advisor for review. This systematic and structured approach to drafting and revising made his overall goal seem more achievable because he could see what he would do step by step. He was also better able to embrace the process of writing and allow himself to write an imperfect first draft because he could see he had time to edit each section. Most of my clients plan 1 to 2 weeks of work at a time with daily goals. At times it is possible to plan only a few days of work at a time because you may need to do some initial work to determine the next steps to take.

For example, it is quite common for my clients to plan 1 to 3 days of literature searching before they can create a reading plan. Once they have located key articles and books they need to read, they list the individual articles and identify which chapters and books they plan to read. Then, using that list, they plan their reading in more detail. In this type of plan, it is usually best to schedule specific readings for specific days. Indicate which book chapters or articles you will read, and if a particular reading is dense and difficult, you can divide it into smaller chunks (e.g., read the first 25 pages in the morning and the second 25 pages in the afternoon). What matters most is that you keep some kind of plan in place so you continue being the project manager of your project.

BENEFITS OF PROJECT MANAGEMENT

The project management approach has many benefits:

1. When you plan ahead what you will do each day, you can spend more energy actually writing and less energy figuring out what you need to do. Such planning helps curb the need to warm up to your work in each writing session.

2. Action plans help you make better use of time; by breaking your goals into small pieces, you can make progress even if you have only short windows of time to work.

3. Your action plan can give you a real sense of accomplishment that so often eludes writers. The reward of earning a degree or being published is so far out in the future that it is easy to end the day feeling as if you are not progressing, regardless of how much you accomplish, because there is still so much more work to do. Dividing your writing goals into small tasks and completing them one at a time also helps you build momentum and experience the sense of accomplishment that comes from crossing tasks off your list.

4. You can use your action plan to plan other aspects of your life in addition to your writing project. For example, many of my clients incorporate into their plan their teaching or other job responsibilities, their job search activities, other types of writing, exercise, family time, social events, and any other goals or responsibilities they have. I also encourage students to deliberately plan time off. You will take that time off, even if you don't plan it, so why not plan ahead and increase your sense of entitlement to taking a break by scheduling rest and meaningful breaks that you need?

When you create an action plan, feel free to experiment with planning other aspects of your life. Planning that accounts for the bigger picture of all that you manage in your life makes it more likely you will set realistic writing goals and actually be able to stick to your writing plan (Miller, 2009).

PROJECT MANAGEMENT GUIDELINES

Four project management guidelines can steer you toward success in your writing project:

1. Set writing goals that are small and specific.
2. Connect each action on your plan to a specific day of the week and perhaps even to a place and a time of day.
3. Plan realistically, and revise your plan when you get off track.
4. Create and maintain your action plans in an electronic format.

> Planning that accounts for the bigger picture of all that you manage in your life makes it more likely you will set realistic writing goals and actually be able to stick to your writing plan.

Set Small and Specific Writing Goals

Set writing goals that are small and specific. Planning to "write Chapter 3," for example, is too big. It is not easily apparent from this description of the task what specific actions to take, how to get started, and what you can reasonably accomplish on a day-to-day basis. Instead, you would be much better off breaking this goal into smaller ones: Create a detailed outline of Chapter 3, draft each outline point or section, and revise and edit each section. As you complete each task, you can experience the pleasure of crossing them off. Many people resist this level of detail and would rather just get to writing instead of spending time planning their writing. In fact, in the long run, planning specific tasks saves you time because you are more likely to work and make use of the time you do have.

Connect Each Action to Logistics

Connect each action on your plan to a specific day of the week and perhaps even to a place you will work and a time of day. Making declarations about what, where (e.g., library, home, coffee shop), and when you will write may make it more likely that you will complete the planned work for that day.

Plan Realistically and Revise

Plan realistically, and revise your plan when you get off track. Do your best to be honest with yourself when you set writing goals. Anxiety and the pressure to perform may disrupt your ability to plan realistically, so plan conservatively. People often feel demoralized when they can't keep up with their own work plans, and they are likely to stop planning altogether when they continually get off track. It can take time to recalibrate and develop a better gauge of what is realistic. I have seen many students develop better planning sensibilities and learn to make more realistic estimates of the time required to complete dissertation and thesis goals. The key is to stick to the project management approach and keep revising your plan regularly, learning from the experience as you go.

You will need to revise your writing plan no matter how good your intentions or how realistic you thought you were when you made the plan. For example, writing a particular section may require more time and effort than you initially realized. Other life responsibilities may take precedence, or you may just have an off day. If you fall behind or get off track, you have a choice: You can beat yourself up, which will only create negative emotions and make procrastination more likely as you seek to avoid those emotions, or you can embrace the reality of where you are and refocus your attention on what you can do now to move forward. I encourage my clients to use the mantra "I am where I am." This mantra reminds you to acknowledge your current reality and refocus your attention on how you can positively move forward.

Aim to spend 15 to 20 minutes at the end of each day being a project manager. Assess where you are, and if the plan for the next day needs to be revised, revise it accordingly. I also encourage you to end each work day by

- Identifying any materials, such as books, articles, a printed draft of your dissertation or thesis, or data analysis output, you will need to meet the next day's goals
- Organizing those materials so they are ready to be used
- Scheduling a start time for writing or zones of writing time in your plan to set the stage for a productive next day.

Use an Electronic Format
Create and maintain your action plans in an electronic format. Students tend to ignore handwritten plans and are generally less motivated to revise and update them. My clients and I use Google Docs, a file-sharing service that is free and accessible to anyone with an Internet connection. It is easy to use (it is basically an open source version of Microsoft Word), and you can learn more about it at www.docs.google.com. The advantages of using this service are that Google Docs are stored remotely (not on your computer), so you can access them from any computer as long as you have an Internet connection, and you can share the documents with one or more people by invitation. Google Docs are password protected, and other people can access them only if invited.

Nearly all of my clients and I share access to their weekly action plans in Google Docs, and we both have the ability to edit the documents. Putting your plan in Google Docs and sharing it with someone else who is willing to regularly check your progress (and, one would hope, leave encouraging notes for you) is a great way to increase your sense of accountability and obtain ongoing support and encouragement to keep writing and move forward.

To help you better understand the project management approach, Table 8.2 provides another example of an action plan. This plan was created by an occupational science doctoral student studying occupation-based motor control practice. The table contains her goals for the week and a

TABLE 8.2. Goals and Action Plan for the Week of October 25

Goals	Date	Action
Write a rough draft of literature review section on occupation-based practice models	Monday October 25	Read and write summary of Kielhofner & Burke (1980) Read and write summary of Lee (2010) review Run 3 miles Spend 30 minutes prepping for Tuesday's class
	Tuesday October 26	7 a.m. yoga class Read and write summary of Chapters 1 and 2 from Kielhofner (2008) Read and write summary of Dunn et al. (1994) Read and write summary of Schkade & Schultz (2003) Teach 5–6:30 p.m.
	Wednesday October 27	Read and write summary of Christiansen & Baum (1991) Read and write summaries for any additional articles from Lee (2010) review Write rough draft of literature review section on occupation-based practice models based on articles read to date Spend 1 hour prepping for Thursday's class
Write a rough draft of literature review section on motor control	Thursday October 28	Run 2–3 miles in morning Read and write summary of Gillen (2005) Read and write summary of Mathiowetz (2004) Draft approximately half of the literature review section on motor control based on articles read to date Teach 5–6:30 p.m.
	Friday October 29	Read and write summary of Wu, Trombly, Lin, & Tickle-Degnen (2000) Draft remaining half of the literature review section on motor control based on articles read to date Grade 5 student reaction papers

(continued)

TABLE 8.2. Goals and Action Plan for the Week of October 25 *(Cont.)*

Goals	Date	Action
	Saturday October 30	Run 2–3 miles in morning
		Read and write summary of Wu, Trombly, Lin, & Tickle-Degnen (1998)
		Read and write summary of Flinn (1995)
		Grade 10 student reaction papers
	Sunday October 31	Integrate literature read Friday and Saturday into draft of literature review section on motor control
		Grade 5 student reaction papers
		Create a new action plan for the week of November 1–7
		Enjoy Halloween!

breakdown of what she planned to do on a daily basis to meet those weekly goals. Her two weekly goals were about creating a rough draft of two sections of her literature review using a subset of the overall literature she planned to read. At this point, she was planning to write both sections at a basic level and expand them later. The smaller actions planned throughout the week collectively enabled her to meet the overall goals. Also, this student planned her exercise schedule and some teaching responsibilities to make sure she was accounting for other important priorities in her life.

CHOICE IN PROJECT MANAGEMENT

In the hectic modern world, it is easy to feel that life has become one long list of things you must do. Your mind may tell you that you must work hard every day, that you should not take much time off, or that you are not accomplishing enough no matter what you do. These kinds of thoughts contribute to the feeling that you don't have full freedom to choose what you do and when you do it.

Yes, it is true that you will not earn a graduate degree or be published if you don't do the necessary work. At the same time, though, you have more choice about what you do day to day than you realize. I support my clients in experiencing a greater sense of choice by using a gas flame metaphor. *Imagine a burner on a gas stove. The burner can be on or off. When it* is on, the flame can be adjusted from high to low. Many of my clients operate as if their only two choices when it comes to dissertation or thesis writing are being on high flame or off. Either they are writing frantically, trying to get as much done as possible, or they are doing very little and avoiding or disengaging from writing.

In reality, you have more choices about how high you set your writing flame. You can deliberately choose to be anywhere from a slow simmer all the way up to a rolling boil. Of course, you can also choose to turn off the burner and deliberately take a break from writing. I encourage you, as part of being a project manager, to consciously choose how high you set your writing flame and to continually assess and adjust the flame on the basis of your progress, timeline, other life roles and responsibilities, and rest and downtime needs.

There are times when high flame is useful (e.g., when a deadline looms), but if you try to write on high flame for long periods, you may burn out. When other responsibilities are competing for your attention, working at a slower, simmer pace is realistic and sustainable. Most of the time, my clients do well to set their flame on low medium or medium. At this level your action plan has some degree of ambition, but you have room to breathe and attend to other areas of life. In the long run, my clients who move between low and medium flame are more productive than those who attempt to operate at high flame day after day. Be conscious of where you set your writing flame, and adjust your plan according to your own needs, the writing you are seeking to do, and your honest intuitive sense of what is realistic for you to accomplish in a given time period.

Managing Your Writing Project

As you write, remember that struggle, procrastination, perfectionism, and difficulty progressing are common, even normal, experiences. The inherent challenges of writing a dissertation can be a great opportunity for you to grow not only professionally but also personally. You can learn to be more aware of your own thoughts and feelings about writing and of ways to move forward when they threaten to hold you back. You can also develop and discover your own writing process that allows you to learn effectively, work consistently, and improve your work over time. Project management skills will benefit you not only as a graduate student but also in your career and life after graduate school.

REFERENCES

Bolker, J. (1998). *Writing your dissertation in fifteen minutes a day*. New York: Henry Holt.

Doctorow, E. L. (1988). *Writers at Work: The Paris Review Interviews* (8th series, George Plimpton, Ed.). New York: Viking.

Dweck, C. S. (2000). *Self-theories: Their role in motivation, personality, and development*. Philadelphia: Psychology Press.

Dweck, C. S. (2002). Beliefs that make smart people dumb. In R. Sternberg (Ed.), *Why smart people can be so stupid* (pp. 24–41). New Haven, CT: Yale University Press.

Dweck, C. S. (2006). *Mindset: The new psychology of success*. New York: Random House.

Eifert, G. H., & Forsyth, J. P. (2005). *Acceptance and commitment therapy for anxiety disorders: A practitioner's guide to using mindfulness, acceptance, and values-based behavior change strategies*. Oakland, CA: New Harbinger.

Hayes, S. C., & Smith, S. (2005). *Get out of your mind and into your life: The new acceptance and commitment therapy*. Oakland, CA: New Harbinger.

Hayes, S. C., Strosahl, K. D., & Wilson, K. G. (1999). *Acceptance and commitment therapy: An experiential approach to behavior change*. New York: Guilford.

Hewitt, P. L., & Flett, G. L. (1991). Perfectionism in the self and social contexts: Conceptualization, assessment, and association with psychopathology. *Journal of Personality and Social Psychology, 60*, 456–470.

Knaus, W. (2002). *The procrastination workbook*. Oakland, CA: New Harbinger.

Lamott, A. (1994). *Bird by bird*. New York: Anchor Books.

Miller, A. B. (2009). *Finish your dissertation once and for all*. Washington, DC: American Psychological Association.

9

Presenting Your Research Findings

CATHERINE FOSTER, BA, and LUTHER G. KALB, MHS

Presenting research is a challenging yet rewarding process that will enable you to continue learning about the field and yourself throughout the course of your career.

—FOSTER AND KALB

One exciting element of the research process is presenting your work to others. While you are hard at work, spending many hours gathering data and crunching numbers at a computer, the knowledge that you will soon share those findings and be recognized for your efforts may be your light at the end of the tunnel. Whether you are building on the work of others or starting a new and exciting endeavor of your own, sharing your efforts leads to increased knowledge in your field.

By disseminating your research findings, you support and build on *evidence-based practice,* or "the conscientious, explicit, and judicious use of current best evidence in making decisions about the care of individual patients" (Sackett, Rosenberg, Muir Gray, Haynes, & Richardson, 1996, p. 71). Moreover, presenting your findings will lead to opportunities to network with other researchers and providers in your field. You may be surprised by how many people are interested in your research topic or have thought of exploring it themselves. Networking and feedback from others can aid in the evolution of your ideas, lead to future research projects, and help make important connections that will further your career.

This chapter provides useful information both for students who have completed a research project for academic credit and wish to share it with a broader audience and for well-seasoned clinicians who are just breaking into the world of research. We describe the process of getting ready to publish a research report, choosing a format and venue for the work, organizing the content of the report, and preparing tables and figures. There are other ways to present your findings, such as seminars, symposia, and workshops (Cleary & Walter, 2004), but this chapter focuses on the poster session, conference presentation, and journal article.

Getting Ready to Publish

Knowing whether or not research is ready for publication requires examining a project with an unbiased eye and review of many factors. In general, the end result of a project that is worthy of publication is due to work done before the project was even begun. A well-planned project will enhance the chances of future publication.

OUTLINING THE RESEARCH QUESTION AND PLAN

Start by outlining the research question and plan in detail. A literature search can show if someone has already published about this same question and the results. Planning the methodology before beginning will decrease the likelihood of glaring methodological errors that would lead to a study not being publishable.

SHARING THE PROJECT WITH OTHERS

After conducting the study and analyzing the results, it is helpful to share the project with others. Colleagues can identify strengths and weaknesses of the project that may help or hinder your chances of publication.

MATCHING THE STUDY TO THE PUBLISHING FORMAT AND VENUE

Whether the project is ready for publication also depends on the publishing format and venue. A study still in a pilot phase may be ready for publication as a poster but not as a paper (see the following section on choosing a format to learn more about this aspect of publication).

COLLABORATING

Collaboration can be a rewarding part of the publication process and can be especially helpful for someone with less experience preparing research for publication (see also Chapter 6 in this volume). An important aspect of collaboration that should be discussed early in the project is the order of authorship.

Typically, authorship is listed in order of study responsibility as well as recognition. The first author typically had the idea for the study and was principally responsible for carrying it out. The second and subsequent authors include everyone who was instrumentally involved in the execution of the study or the manuscript. They may have gathered data, overseen the analysis, or contributed substantially to the content of the manuscript.

Sometimes the last author is the "senior" or "anchor" author (e.g., someone with expertise in the area of research) who provided expert review of the manuscript and assisted in responding to reviewer comments. Authors who have contributed equally can be listed alphabetically.

COMMUNICATING THE RESULTS INFORMALLY

An easy and unintimidating way to start the process of communicating research results to others is through informal talks or write-ups. Ways to share research before official submission include providing a lunch-and-learn presentation at work or to fellow students at college, sharing a draft of the research article, or giving a PowerPoint presentation on the study. Asking people who are not heavily involved with the study to review the report with an unbiased eye not only provides constructive feedback but also can help prepare you for the peer review process or the question-and-answer session following a conference presentation.

Informal reviewers will catch flaws and help you generate new thoughts. Use the valuable feedback and insights garnered from them.

SHARING THE FINAL PRODUCT

Once you are comfortable that you have captured all relevant suggestions, choose a format and venue to disseminate the final product. Many works

> **Which format is best for communicating your study to others depends on what stage the study is in and how expansive the information is.**

are available that review the publication process in more depth; see Cooper (2010) and Lester (2012) for more information.

Choosing a Format

Which format is best for communicating your study to others depends on what stage the study is in and how expansive the information is. A pilot study or study that has generated only preliminary data may be best disseminated in a conference poster. If the study is complete and all data are gathered and analyzed, consider submitting a full conference presentation or journal article. A case study may be best presented in a poster, whereas a study with a larger number of participants (thus more data and stronger results) may be best for a conference presentation or article. The scholarly level, referring to the quality of the study, including the methodology, professional writing style, and whether the research has been previously published, is also important.

As always, there are exceptions. Pilot studies do get written up in journals, just as case studies may be shared through conference presentations. At times, the presentation format may be decided for you. For instance, conference organizers may accept an abstract and then ask you to submit either a poster or full presentation. If you were hoping to do a presentation but your abstract is accepted as a poster, it is still worth taking advantage of the opportunity to share your work with others (Cleary & Walter, 2004). For more information on this topic, see Browner (2012).

POSTERS

Posters are most frequently displayed at conferences, although they may also be presented elsewhere, such as at a research symposium for graduate students in their department. One might choose to do a poster for many reasons. Posters typically are not at the same scholarly level as journal articles and will not undergo as rigorous a peer review process. A poster session makes information available faster than a journal article, which may take a year or more to reach the public (Cleary & Walter, 2004). Also, a poster allows you to directly interact with people who are interested in your research.

Informing others of your investigation face to face can be both exciting *and* anxiety provoking. If you have not presented before, you may want to start with a poster, which is more casual and less stressful than a conference presentation in front of a large audience (Taggart & Arslanian, 2000). Chapter 15 in this book provides more advice on presenting effectively in person.

The poster process starts with a brief abstract being submitted that goes through a peer review process before being accepted. Because of the time lag between when an abstract is submitted and a poster is presented, the poster may have slightly different results than the abstract if you have collected more data in the interim. Typically displayed on a large (e.g., 4 ft. by 6 ft.), flat poster board or laminated paper, posters display a summary of a research study. Many options are available online for having a poster professionally printed.

Much of a poster's effectiveness depends on aesthetics. How a poster looks will influence whether someone stops to read the text. A good start is to have a title that is intriguing but not so unusual that no one will be able to determine what the study is about. Most posters follow a general layout for presenting information (see Figure 9.1; the contents of each section are discussed in more detail later in this chapter). Where appropriate, replacing words with graphs, tables, and pictures can break up the text and liven up the layout.

Generally, in poster sessions at conferences, many posters (sometimes hundreds) are displayed at once, with hundreds of people milling about the display area. Presenting a poster allows you to share your research through an engaging one-on-one experience with a wide variety of people, and their feedback can help you gain new insights and make connections in the field (have business cards and a sign-up sheet so you can e-mail a copy of your poster later to interested attendees).

You likely will have each audience member's attention only for a short time. Many conference goers want a quick snapshot of a study instead of reading the whole poster. You should have ready a brief presentation touching on the main points of each section of the poster (especially any graphics). Your goal is to draw people in and engage them before they move on to another poster.

Once you get people talking, it is much easier to maintain their attention, especially by asking them about their own research interests. This is the

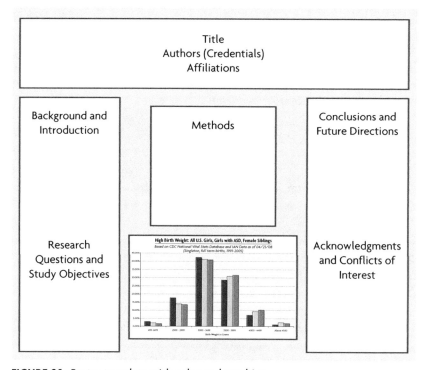

FIGURE 9.1. Poster template with color and graphics.

satisfying part! A poster can be an effective way to communicate your research to a mass audience, and it gives you a chance to practice explaining your research, face to face, to others (Cleary & Walter, 2004).

A poster can also be a launching point for taking a study to the next level of publication. Many studies that become printed journal articles are first presented as a poster. A poster can be built upon to later submit to a journal.

What may be most important is to engage the audience in the moment. Anticipate prospective questions, and prepare some responses ahead of time. For instance, preparing some talking points about the more confusing aspects of the study (such as a complicated statistical procedure

> **What may be most important is to engage the audience in the moment. Anticipate prospective questions, and prepare some responses ahead of time.**

that is beyond what most researchers use), an important limitation, or a conclusion that has been drawn, is crucial to a high-quality presentation. Preparing for likely questions or criticisms is a useful tactic to avoid being flustered and to improve your confidence during the actual presentation.

CONFERENCE PRESENTATIONS

Conference presentations (or oral talks) are often reserved for complete and high-quality studies. Typically, a conference has many more posters presented than conference talks, and thus it is usually more prestigious to have an abstract accepted as a conference presentation after it has gone through the peer review process. Some conferences allow you to choose whether you are submitting your abstract for either presentation method, or you may be able to select only one.

Typically, a conference presentation involves one person orally presenting a study in detail to a large seated audience. Presentations also may be in a panel format of multiple speakers who are experts on a specified topic. Presenters typically use graphics or videos in a PowerPoint presentation.

As with poster presentations, practice and timing are key, and preparation for probable questions from the audience will lead to a more seamless presentation (again, see Chapter 15 for tips on presenting to an audience). If the talk is timed, prepare in advance to avoid racing through information. Practice your talk to be sure it is the proper length, and identify your "key" and "cut" sections. If you find yourself running out of time, highlight the key sections and go over the cut sections quickly (or skip them entirely). Close with a "take-home message"—that is, the most important point you want to convey to the audience.

JOURNAL ARTICLES

Journal articles require the greatest detail and command the highest quality of work. Journals are typically interested in studies that present new, original results or methods; reinterpret or refine previous research; or summarize the present knowledge around a subject. Journal articles are also expected to be useful, clearly written, thoroughly researched (including citations), and logically developed. If your project meets these considerations, is methodologically sound, and contributes to a better understanding of a problem, then consider submitting it for publication.

Choosing an appropriate journal is critical to successfully publishing a study. Because you can submit to only one journal at a time, make sure that the article is a good fit. Most journals provide author guidelines for submissions, list topics of interest to the journal, give the journal's ranking (the *impact factor*), and explain publication policies. For additional questions, contact the journal's editorial office or editorial board. For more information about how to write and where to publish an article, see Nahata (2008) and Chernick (2012).

In a peer-reviewed journal, each study is reviewed for quality by several (usually two to four) reviewers with expertise in the relevant field, who recommend whether to publish as is, reject, or request either minor or significant revisions. Reviewers often do request revisions, and once the requested changes are made, the article goes through the submission process again. If the reviewers or editor-in-chief finds that you have addressed the requests adequately, the article is formally accepted for publication.

Depending on the publication, the article may be professionally copyedited. Typically you have the opportunity to review the copyediting and answer any queries about the clarity of the language, study details, or data presented. You also may see page proofs of your article just before it is published. Although the process can take weeks or months and may involve substantial additional work, having your article edited by experts on the topic usually substantially improves your contribution to the literature. For more information on preparing an article for submission, see the American Psychological Association (APA; 2010a, 2010b); Samset (1999); and Shidham, Pitman, and DeMay (2012).

Organizing the Content

Regardless of format, a research study is typically organized into six sections:

1. Abstract
2. Introduction and literature review
3. Methods
4. Results
5. Discussion and conclusion
6. References.

For more information see, for example, APA (2010b).

ABSTRACT

The abstract is the first narrative about a study that readers encounter. We recommend writing this section last, however, because a succinct distillation of a study's key aspects is difficult to accomplish until the end of the writing process. The abstract, as well as the title, should be clear, concise, and convey the core purpose and findings of your work.

The APA (2010b) optimum word length for an abstract is 150–250 words to sum up all important points. Do not include citations or repeat the title, and instead of using "I" or "we," use the active, third-person voice, such as "the study shows" or "the researchers suggest." The abstract should answer the questions, Why was this study done? What did you do, and how? What results did you find? What do these findings mean?

INTRODUCTION AND LITERATURE REVIEW

The introduction sets the stage for the study. The opening or thesis paragraph should clearly convey the problem and put the topic in perspective. Although the problem statement itself is usually a single sentence, it is accompanied by several paragraphs that provide the scope and depth of the problem. These paragraphs provide the rationale for the research, including why the problem is important, how the study relates to broader and more important issues, and how the study either fills a particular gap or overcomes inadequacies in prior research.

The introduction also includes a review of previous research or relevant literature (see Chapter 10 in this volume on conducting a literature review). This review shows what previous research has (or has not) accomplished and concludes by describing the clarity your research brings to the subject. The length and depth of this part of the introduction depend on how much research has previously been done in the area.

The literature review should focus on and cite recent empirical or peer-reviewed studies. Less rigorous research, editorials, and Internet blogs, for example, are usually not appropriate in a research report.

The introduction also can describe the conceptual framework or theoretical model your study is based on—that is, the set of ideas or theories that organizes, grounds, and explains your research. Define all important terms, especially those unique to your field or unfamiliar to readers. At the end of the introduction, a single statement or paragraph explains what you intended to accomplish in the study, including your hypotheses.

METHODS

The methods section describes the study design and how you carried out the research. The methods must directly relate to the research questions and conceptual framework, as well as to the statistical plan for each research question. The following sections cover (1) population and sampling, (2) instruments, (3) procedures, and (4) data analysis.

Population and Sampling

The population and sampling subsection describes the population from which the participants were gathered and the methods for recruiting participants (e.g., from a local hospital, online), inclusion and exclusion criteria (i.e., characteristics of people allowed and not allowed to participate in the study), and criteria for dividing participants into groups (e.g., control vs. experimental conditions or randomized vs. nonrandomized allocation).

If appropriate, describe how previous research informed the sampling methodology. For instance, did other authors find a problem with including particular age groups or recommend using an approach different from previous ones? Report the demographic characteristics of the sample, including age (often expressed as a mean and range); gender; socioeconomic status (e.g., education level, family income); and other characteristics of the sample (e.g., race, ethnicity), as appropriate. Demographic data also can be reported in a table or figure.

Instruments

In most research, either observational or experimental, the researcher uses some type of survey or questionnaire, stimulus, or measurement to gather data. The instruments section is a brief description of the questionnaire, its development, and the reasons it was chosen for the study. Provide data from the developer on the measure's consistency (i.e., *reliability*) and ability to measure what it is supposed to (i.e., *validity*). Cite each instrument and any literature that guided your decision-making process in the reference list.

Procedures

The procedures section states exactly what you did—how you carried out the experiment, any special procedures followed, how you collected the data (including a description of what data are missing), and so forth. You also should describe in detail the consent procedures you used, including how many participants agreed to the study terms (e.g., prospective benefits, risks) and specify the institutional review board that approved the project. This section should have enough detail and clarity to allow others to replicate the study.

Data Analysis

State what variables were included in the data analyses, particularly the dependent and independent variables, and what statistical tests were chosen and why. Specify the decision-making criteria (e.g., the critical alpha level or p value) and any other statistics used in answering the research question.

Although discussion of the most appropriate statistics is beyond the scope of this chapter, some commonly reported statistics include t, F, and chi-square values, as well as regression parameters, effect sizes, and p values. These values must be accompanied by appropriate descriptive statistics, such as confidence intervals, mean or median scores, R^2 values, and so forth. Be sure to explain how these values are connected to your findings and conclusions.

Also specify the computer software you used for the analysis. Programs such as SPSS (SPSS, Chicago) and SAS (SAS Institute, Cary, NC) are used for management, graphing, and analysis of data. Microsoft Excel, which is more user-friendly, has excellent graphing features and can perform some statistical analyses, but it is limited for data management. For more information on data analysis, see the University of California at Los Angeles Statistical Consulting Group's (n.d.) Web site, a free resource of seminars, textbooks, and examples that are illustrated across a variety of statistical software programs.

RESULTS

The results section describes the study's findings and includes specific data and statistics. When writing the results section, always consult the relevant style manual for any specific instructions for formatting this section. Present lengthy series of data in a table or figure, and direct readers to each at the appropriate point in the text (e.g., "see Table 1"). All tables and figures must have a number and a descriptive title; more detail on communicating data in tables and figures is provided later in this chapter.

DISCUSSION AND CONCLUSION

The discussion section summarizes findings, gives conclusions about their meaning, and highlights clinical or research implications. Briefly reflect on how the study expanded on the current body of literature and whether the findings were different from those found in previous studies. If they are different, explain why.

Identify the limitations of the study, which include potential shortcomings in the study's design (e.g., small sample size), and also highlight any strengths. Finally, discuss future directions for related research, such as use of a different approach or ways to strengthen or expand on the study's findings.

REFERENCES

Every journal provides clear rules for how to cite and reference a source (e.g., the *American Journal of Occupational Therapy* uses APA style [APA, 2010b]; see also Chapter 7 in this book). The manuscript must conform to these policies to be considered for publication. We recommend reference management software such as RefWorks or EndNote to ease this process given there are many reference styles. See the journal's author guidelines or style manual before developing the references section.

Communicating Data in Tables and Graphs

The visual display of data is an effective way to convey information. There are many ways to present data graphically, and the effort involved in selecting and preparing the right one will pay off in the increased effectiveness of your report. Tables and figures (figures include charts, graphs, and photos; this discussion focuses on graphs) are often used in reporting the results of a research study because, when appropriately designed, they convey complex information quickly and clearly, allowing you to avoid a lengthy narrative description of your study's results. However, many journals limit the amount of display materials in an article, so be sure to consult the author guidelines before developing many figures or tables.

> Tables and figures ...
> convey complex information
> quickly and clearly.

TABLES

Tables can be the best way to present data and should be carefully developed with the same attention to detail as text. Tables are most commonly used to summarize lengthy, complex information about the study such as statistical results or descriptive information about the sample. Each table requires a title (column, row, and overall table title), explanation of abbreviations in footnotes, and is usually numbered and cited in sequence in the text. See Table 9.1 as an example.

TABLE 9.1. Demographic Information, by Group

Demographic	% ASD ($n = 55$)	% ADHD ($n = 24$)
Age, years	$M = 10.3, SD = 2.9$	$M = 9.3, SD = 2.1$
Sex: male	87	100
Handedness: Right	84	75
Parent education: High school	5	13
Parent education: Some college	27	21
Parent education: Post college	33	17

Note. ASD = autism spectrum disorder; ADHD = attention deficit hyperactivity disorder.

GRAPHS

Graphs have the unique ability to demonstrate complex concepts, such as time-series trends, interaction effects, and distributions, that would be cumbersome to communicate in words. Graphs are appropriate for quantitative data, or numerical values.

Two types of quantitative data are used in graphs: (1) *continuous data,* which have a range of values, and (2) *discrete data,* which have a finite number of possible values. For example, physiological measurements (e.g., heart rate, body mass index) would take on a range of values, constituting a continuous variable. Data pertaining to successful completion of a task such as putting on shoes or eating a meal may take on a "yes" or "no" value, representing a binary or discrete value.

For quantitative data, one must consider how the data were measured. For instance, is the outcome, otherwise known as the *dependent variable,* time, a count, or a score? Considering the nature of the data is of premier importance when selecting your graph. Choosing the most appropriate graph, given a set of data, is discussed in further detail below.

We recommend following these guidelines when preparing a graph:

- Label graphs clearly, and use a simple design. Avoid cluttering a graph with unnecessary lines, colors, or patterns.
- Make the graph relevant to the subject. Unnecessary graphs take up space and dilute the quality of the presentation.
- Develop the graph so that it is completely self-explanatory. All necessary labels should be clear, and all abbreviations should be spelled out in either the body of the graph or a footnote.

Figure 9.2 details the information required for readers to interpret a graph done for a study on attendance rates in an outpatient autism clinic over an 18-month period. These vital elements include a figure caption,

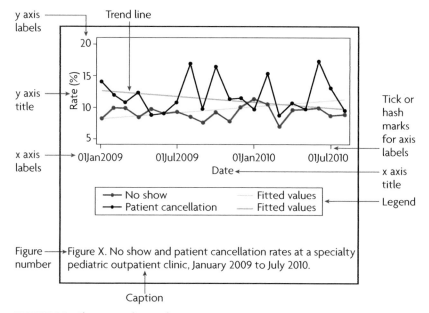

FIGURE 9.2. Elements of a graph.

titles for the *x* (horizontal) and *y* (vertical) axes, a label and tick mark for each value on the axes, and a legend for interpreting any patterns or colors.

The sections that follow describe the most commonly used graphs for portraying research results. See Nichol and Pexman (2010) and Freeman, Walters, and Campbell (2008) for more detailed explanations of the best ways to graphically represent data.

Pie Graphs

Pie graphs are a simple way to display the size of each portion relative to the whole (100%). Pie graphs are easy to interpret, but they show only one type of data.

All slices should indicate the variable they represent and the percentage (totaling 100). Each slice should be separated or clearly discernible; too many slices (e.g., more than 6 or 8) make the pie graph difficult to interpret. The largest slice begins at the top of the graph (i.e., 12 o'clock) and is followed by the other segments in order of descending size. Figure 9.3 shows the gender distribution of participants in an autism study, clearly highlighting that most were male.

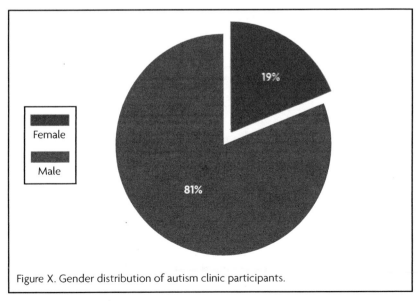

Figure X. Gender distribution of autism clinic participants.

FIGURE 9.3. Pie graph.

Line Graphs and Scatter Plots

A line graph or scatter plot is a relatively simple way to illustrate how two or more variables are related. Both scatter plots and line graphs are useful in studies that measure a variable over time and in correlational analyses. Often, these graphs are used to represent change in an outcome (*dependent variable*) as a function of an intervention (*independent variable*).

Line graphs are simply data points connected by lines. Figure 9.4 shows the decrease over time in the percentage of clients who had medical assistance at an outpatient pediatric clinic.

Scatter plots have many dots, each representing a relationship between two variables. Dots that cluster around a line, for example, show that the variables are related, whereas those scattered at random are not related. A trend line can be added to the plot to express an average trend. Figure 9.5 depicts the relationship or a positive correlation between internalizing (e.g., depression and anxiety) and externalizing (e.g., behavior problems) symptoms of children participating in an autism study.

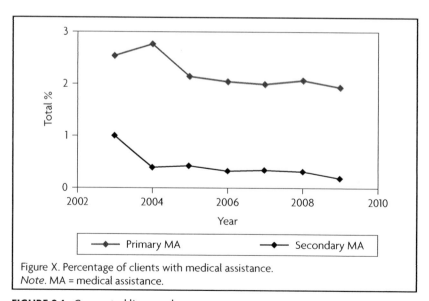

Figure X. Percentage of clients with medical assistance.
Note. MA = medical assistance.

FIGURE 9.4. Connected line graph.

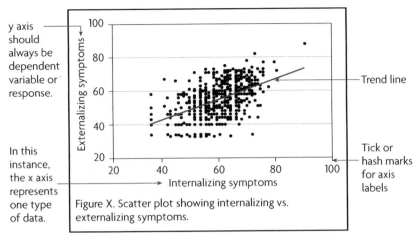

FIGURE 9.5. Scatter plot with trend lines.

Bar Charts

In a *bar chart*, rectangular bars (either vertical or horizontal) show the relative size of the values they represent. Bar charts can be used for plotting both discrete and continuous data.

A bar chart allows readers to easily compare groups of data, but as with pie graphs, their usefulness in displaying relationships or complex data is limited. Figure 9.6 shows trends in new and total clients seen at an outpatient autism center between 2004 and 2009.

Distribution Graphs

Distribution graphs, such as histograms and box-and-whisker plots, are used to illustrate frequency distributions (i.e., displaying a count of data).

In histograms, the height of the bars represents an observed frequency, the *x* axis represents the category of data, and the *y* axis shows the frequency or actual count of the data (see Figure 9.7, which shows the distribution of pediatric mental health scores of children enrolled in an autism study). A smoothed curve is overlaid to assist with visualization.

A *box plot,* also known as a *box-and-whisker diagram,* is a convenient way to graphically depict groups of data through a 5-point summary that includes the smallest observations or lower quartile (Q1, bottom 25%),

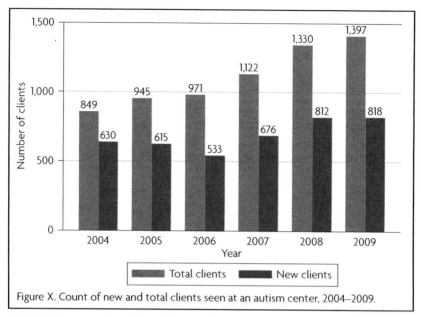

Figure X. Count of new and total clients seen at an autism center, 2004–2009.

FIGURE 9.6. Bar graph with trend lines and ranges.

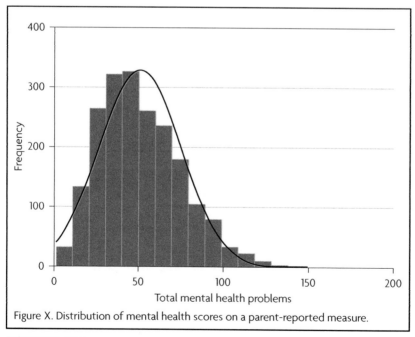

Figure X. Distribution of mental health scores on a parent-reported measure.

FIGURE 9.7. Histogram.

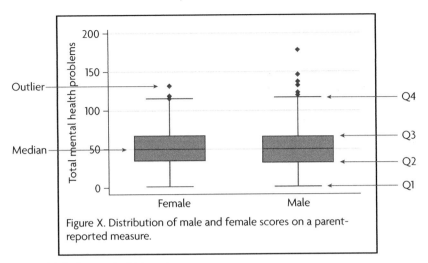

FIGURE 9.8. Box-and-whisker plot.

median (Q2, 50%), and upper quartile (Q3, 75%; see Figure 9.8). The spacings between the different parts of the boxes help indicate the degree of dispersion *(spread)* and skewness in the data. The top and bottom bars (or *whiskers*) reflect the range. When there is an observation outside of the quartiles, this represents an unusually large (or small) observation, otherwise known as an *outlier*.

Box plots can be drawn either horizontally or vertically (see Rosner [1995] for further details). Figure 9.8 presents the same information as Figure 9.7, except the data in Figure 9.8 are stratified by gender.

Presenting Your Findings

Preparing for a presentation of research forces you to reexamine your work from concept to conclusion, an important part of the learning process. You do not have to be a seasoned researcher to add your contribution to the many conferences and journals that disseminate research findings. In the end, the process of sharing research is both personally rewarding and an invaluable contribution to the occupational therapy profession's knowledge base.

REFERENCES

American Psychological Association. (2010a). *Preparing manuscripts for publication in psychology journals: A guide for new authors.* Available online at http://www.apa.org/pubs/authors/new-author-guide.pdf

American Psychological Association. (2010b). *Publication manual of the American Psychological Association* (6th ed.). Washington, DC: Author.

Browner, W. S. (2012). *Publishing and presenting clinical research* (3rd ed.). Philadelphia: Lippincott Williams & Wilkins.

Chernick, V. (2012). How to get your paper accepted for publication. *Paediatric Respiratory Review, 13*(2), 130–132.

Cleary, M., & Walter, G. (2004). Apportioning our time and energy: Oral presentation, poster, journal article, or other? *International Journal of Mental Health Nursing, 13,* 204–207.

Cooper, L. (2010). *Reporting research in psychology: How to meet journal article reporting standards.* Washington, DC: American Psychological Association.

Freeman, J., Walters, S., & Campbell, M. (2008). *How to display data.* Hoboken, NJ: Wiley.

Lester, J. D. (2012). *Writing research papers: A complete guide* (14th ed.). White Plains, NY: Longman.

Nahata, M. C. (2008). Tips for writing and publishing an article. *Annals of Pharmacotherapy, 42*(3), 273–277.

Nichol, A., & Pexman, P. (2010). *Displaying your findings: A practical guide for creating figures, posters, and presentations.* Washington, DC: American Psychological Association.

Rosner, B. (1995). *Fundamentals of biostatistics.* Pacific Grove, CA: Duxbury Press.

Sackett, D., Rosenberg, W., Muir Gray, J. A., Haynes, R. B., & Richardson, W. S. (1996). Evidence-based medicine: What it is and what it isn't. *British Medical Journal, 312,* 71. Retrieved September 12, 2011, from http://www.bmj.com/content/312/7023/71.full

Samset, J. (1999). Dear author—Advice from a retiring editor. *American Journal of Epidemiology, 150*(5), 432–436.

Shidham, V., Pitman, M., & DeMay, R. (2012). How to write an article: Preparing a publishable manuscript! *CytoJournal, 9*(1).

Taggart, H. M., & Arslanian, C. (2000). Creating an effective poster presentation. *Orthopaedic Nursing, 19,* 47–49, 52.

University of California at Los Angeles, Statistical Consulting Group. (n.d.). *Statistical computing.* Available online at http://www.ats.ucla.edu/stat/overview.htm

Writing Systematic Reviews

MARIAN ARBESMAN, PhD, OTR/L

How do you know that what you do and how you do it really works?
—Margo B. Holm (2000)

The amount of research available at any given moment is overwhelming. Whether one is searching the Internet, reading the published literature, or listening to an in-person lecture, the selection from which to choose is enormous, and the quality is variable. Health care professionals and consumers need access to reliable information on research findings, and systematic reviews fill this need. The authors of systematic reviews locate the available studies, categorize them, and summarize the results for readers.

For the biomedical, education, and social sciences literatures, two types of systematic reviews are generally written. The first and most familiar type is the narrative literature review. Narrative reviews have a broad focus, and although the articles included in the review may be of good quality, the author decides which studies to include or exclude and may or may not specify the methodology he or she used to select articles (Collins & Fauser, 2005). The author takes an individualized approach to what the narrative review covers, how it is focused, what databases are used to find information, and how the results are structured. As a result of this nonsystematic and individualized approach, the narrative literature review may include articles in a limited area and may not incorporate the universe of articles covering a given topic.

The systematic review, in contrast, derives its name from the scientific process used to develop a focused question, gather information, classify the information, and determine what the results of the review mean (Cook, Sackett, & Spitzer, 1995). It is an outgrowth of evidence-based practice (EBP), an approach to effective health care delivery that took root in the early 1990s.

According to Law and Baum (1998), in *evidence-based occupational therapy practice* the practitioner "uses research evidence together with clinical knowledge and reasoning to make decisions about interventions that are effective for a specific client" (p. 131). An evidence-based perspective is based on the assumption that one can judge the scientific evidence of an intervention's effectiveness to be more or less strong and valid according to a hierarchy of research designs and an assessment of the quality of the research. Although EBP has been spurred on by the demands of payers, regulators, and consumers, occupational therapists and occupational therapy assistants have been equally eager to provide effective services that are client centered, supported by evidence, and delivered in an efficient and cost-effective manner.

At the same time, many occupational therapy practitioners find it difficult to understand how to use the best available evidence to inform their practice. Many did not acquire critical appraisal skills while in school; others acquired the skills but are not confident in using them. For these practitioners, reviewing the practice-oriented literature on their own is a challenge. In addition, limited access to electronic databases and system-level constraints such as lack of time and management support further limit practitioners' ability to search, retrieve, and appraise evidence from the published literature that could be useful to their practice. Occupational therapy practitioners look to quality systematic reviews for summaries of evidence that are useful for their areas of practice.

Many occupational therapy practitioners find it difficult to understand how to use the best available evidence to inform their practice.

Writing systematic reviews makes a difference by providing important information to clinicians, researchers, educators, and students looking for high-quality summaries of evidence. Systematic reviews are a useful form of research for occupational therapy practitioners interested in analyzing and appraising literature from disparate fields. Occupational therapy researchers may undertake the systematic review process because it provides the opportunity to carry out a rigorous and creative research project without some of the challenges of clinical and laboratory research. For example, a researcher may work at an institution that lacks space for a lab or a client population, or he or she may lack sufficient time to complete the institutional steps required for a clinical project (e.g., obtaining the approval of an institutional review board).

Developing a Focused Question

All types of research begin with a question, and systematic reviews are no exception. According to Tickle-Degnen (1999), systematic review questions typically fall into three categories: descriptive, assessment, and intervention.

Descriptive questions address a diagnosis, clinical condition, or specific patient population. Descriptive questions ask what attributes and outcomes typify particular client populations, their daily lives, and their occupational performance. Questions in this category may ask, What are the effects of visual impairment and age on driving? or Are there differences in play performance between children with versus without sensory processing disorders?

Assessment questions seek to identify the most reliable and valid methods for assessing occupational performance in a specific clinical population. Examples of this type of question might be, What are the most reliable measures for assessing the instrumental activities of daily living performance of community-based elders? and Is a given variable valid for assessing changes in social participation for adults with serious and persistent mental illness? Assessment questions may ask, Are we measuring the specific variable in the most valid and reliable manner? If not, can we develop a better assessment measure?

Intervention questions ask which occupational therapy interventions are most effective in achieving desired outcomes with specific types of clinical conditions and populations. An intervention question might ask, What occupational therapy interventions are effective in the rehabilitation of persons with work-related injuries or with clinical conditions of the hand, wrist, and forearm? High-quality intervention questions are often developed in partnerships between academics and clinicians (Lin, Murphy, & Robinson, 2010).

Focused questions typically pertain to interventions because the major purpose of evidence-based practice is to inform and guide clinical decision making. Targeting descriptive and assessment questions, however, is also valuable to evidence-based practice. Reviews with descriptive questions provide an in-depth understanding of a particular aspect of a population or clinical condition useful for targeting an intervention to a subset of a group. Assessment questions help researchers and practitioners understand which measures are appropriate to use when conducting and evaluating studies or assessing clients.

Intervention and assessment questions typically follow the PICO format (Institute of Medicine, 2008), which ensures that they are clinically relevant and practical for the occupational therapy process. PICO is an acronym that represents four components of the question:

1. P—*participants, population, and problem*—describes who or what the question is about. This component includes the diagnostic criteria, participant characteristics (e.g., age, race, ethnicity), and setting of interest (e.g., community, hospital, outpatient rehabilitation). Defining inclusion and exclusion criteria for the participants, population, and problem streamlines the systematic review process (the focused question may or may not list all of these criteria, as appropriate).

2. I—*intervention*—describes the details of the intervention or therapy being examined and specifies the boundaries of treatment. For example, a reviewer examining the effectiveness of sensory integration for adults with serious mental illness needs to define what studies under the umbrella of sensory integration to include and exclude. Will the review be limited to studies that maintain fidelity to occupational therapy using a sensory integration approach, or will it also include sensory-based interventions? Besides the scope of the therapy being considered, incorporating the duration or frequency of therapy into the focused question may be appropriate.

3. Depending on the research designs included in the review, C—*comparison groups*—may or may not be a consideration. Systematic reviews may be limited to studies that include a comparison group that does not receive intervention. The comparison group may receive standard or usual care, no treatment, or some sort of placebo that mimics parts of the intervention process (e.g., participants in the control group receive the same amount of attention as participants in the intervention group).

4. O—*outcomes of interest*—must be clinically relevant and appropriate. Research studies often contain numerous outcome measures to ensure that all the potential effects of an intervention are considered. Appropri-

ate outcomes may address occupational performance and participation, body structure and function, or any other variable of concern to occupational therapy practitioners.

Two examples of review questions in the PICO format are as follows: (1) For clients with dementia and their caregivers (P), does occupational therapy (I), when compared with no intervention (C), improve daily functioning in clients and sense of competence in caregivers (O)? (2) For children and adolescents with autism spectrum disorder and their families (P), does occupational therapy (I), when compared with no intervention (C), improve performance in school, home, and community occupations (O)? Some focused questions do not include either a comparison group or specific outcome measures—for example, if multiple outcome measures and a variety of study designs are included in the search or if the review author is examining a broad scope of the available literature. An example of this type of question is, For adults with serious mental illness (P), what occupational therapy interventions in the areas of paid and unpaid employment and education (I) are effective?

Establishing a Protocol

A cornerstone of the systematic review is the development of a protocol that outlines the steps involved in the process (Wright, Brand, Dunn, & Spindler, 2007). Although the reviewer may make minimal modifications as the review proceeds, the goals of the protocol are to establish consistency and to allow other researchers to replicate the review. The protocol specifies the literature search methods, the criteria for screening articles for inclusion, and procedures for extracting and analyzing the data. A protocol helps reduce the bias that can occur in narrative reviews (Murphy, Robinson, & Lin, 2009). The protocol should be documented and consulted frequently during the review process.

A systematic review can be labor intensive, and the work can be completed more quickly if other people are involved (see Chapter 6, this volume, on collaboration). Assigning each team member a specific component of the review facilitates the process.

A team approach also promotes quality control; from the development of the focused question to the final summary of results, personal perspective determines what literature to include in a review, how to interpret that literature, and which literature to highlight in the final summary. At each step in the process, one team member may view things differently from another. For example, team members may differ on the assigned level of evidence for an article or may also differ on how to interpret the results of a study. Although any researcher relies to some extent on personal perspective, having others review one's choices results in a more complete product and prevents the review from being too narrow, too broad, or off track. In many systematic reviews, two people review each article when determining inclusion and exclusion, and if they cannot achieve consensus, a third person breaks the tie.

Devising a Search Strategy

The search strategy consists of criteria that will determine the results of the search. General criteria may include the years the search will cover, the languages that can be considered, and the type of research to include (e.g., peer-reviewed literature only, research reports, conference proceedings, nonpublished research). Question-specific criteria might determine, for example, whether all persons with a given diagnosis are included in the review. At this stage in the process, it is also important to consider whether to include studies conducted by professionals other than occupational therapy practitioners but within the scope of occupational therapy practice. Building on what already exists in the occupational therapy literature, studies from other disciplines are useful when the occupational therapy literature for a given topic is limited or the authors wish to offer a broader and potentially less insular perspective on the topic.

DATABASE SELECTION

One goal of a systematic review is to be comprehensive, and it is important to search not only the databases that have important resources for addressing the focused question but also those that marginally touch on the question. Each database provides a slightly different slant on the literature, so incorporating results from all of them provides a comprehensive overview of the available research. Databases are discussed in more detail later in this chapter.

Depending on the researcher's comfort in searching the literature and the time allocated to complete the searches, he or she may consider consulting with a research librarian who has experience in completing systematic reviews. These librarians are familiar with the many available databases and with the filters that can be used to narrow the search results to a manageable quantity (Edward G. Miner Library, n.d.).

SEARCH TERMS

To develop appropriate search terms, the PICO components of the focused question are a good place to start. Consider the question, For adults with serious mental illness (P), what occupational therapy interventions in the areas of paid and unpaid employment and education (I) are effective? Search terms are needed to capture the following:

- Diagnoses and clinical conditions that would fit under the designation of *serious mental illness*. For example, would a study of newly diagnosed adults with schizophrenia be appropriate for the review?
- Parameters of *paid and unpaid employment*. Should *child care, volunteering,* and *continuing education programs* be included in the search in addition to *work, job, employment,* and *vocation*? If so, these terms and any possible synonyms should be used in the search.
- Interventions considered to be within the scope of occupational therapy interventions. Is the review focusing on a specific intervention or all interventions?

Each database serves a unique community of users with its own professional jargon, and the meanings ascribed to a given term may vary widely among disciplines. For example, for an occupational therapy practitioner the term *habit* may conjure up images of a client moving toward greater participation by establishing habits that make it easier to take part in meaningful occupations. Other disciplines view *habits* as behaviors the client needs to change or break, such as smoking cigarettes, drinking alcohol, or shopping excessively. This different perspective becomes evident when searching for literature in PsycINFO versus OTseeker, for example.

Performing the Search

For those with access to a hospital, college, or university library, accessing multiple databases is a simple process, because many libraries subscribe to a wide range of electronic journals. Others without access to these resources may have to look elsewhere to find the databases. Some college and university alumni associations offer online library access as a benefit of association membership, and some occupational therapy academic programs offer library access for practitioners serving as fieldwork supervisors.

SEARCHING DATABASES FOR CITATIONS AND ABSTRACTS

The following bibliographic databases are available for free on the Internet:

- Campbell Collaboration (www.campbellcollaboration.org)
- Cochrane Collaboration (www.cochrane.org)
- Education Resources Information Center (ERIC; www.eric.ed.gov)
- Google Scholar (http://scholar.google.com)
- OTseeker (www.otseeker.com)
- PsycBITE (a database of interventions for persons with brain injuries; http://www.psycbite.com)
- PubMed (www.ncbi.nlm.nih.gov/pubmed).

Members of the American Occupational Therapy Association (AOTA) have access to these databases through the *Evidence-Based Practice Resource Directory* in the "Evidence-Based Practice and Research" section of the AOTA Web site (AOTA, n.d.).

LOCATING FULL-TEXT ARTICLES

Free access to electronic journal articles has been made easier thanks to the Open Access movement, which was first proposed by researchers in the 1960s and became a reality in the 1990s with the advent of technology that allowed for easy compilation and sharing of information (e.g., the Internet, electronic databases, markup language such as HTML). This movement has advocated the unrestricted dissemination of all scientific information (Suber, 2004).

One can access the full text of journal articles through a variety of sources. AOTA members have free access to all archived articles in the *American Journal of Occupational Therapy (AJOT),* the *British Journal of Occupational Therapy,* and the *Canadian Journal of Occupational Therapy.* In addition, those certified through the National Board for Certification in Occupational Therapy have access to ProQuest. PubMed, a service of the

U.S. National Library of Medicine and the National Institutes of Health (NIH), manages PubMed Central, a digital archive of the peer-reviewed biomedical and life science literature (www.pubmedcentral.nih.gov/). The "Journal List" (link is on the home page) shows journals that have articles available for free, including *American Journal of Public Health, BMJ,* and *Occupational and Environmental Medicine* (NIH, 2012).

> **Free access to electronic journal articles has been made easier thanks to the Open Access movement, which was first proposed by researchers in the 1960s and became a reality in the 1990s with the advent of technology that allowed for easy compilation and sharing of information.**

The ERIC database (www.eric.ed.gov) also provides free access to selected journal articles. Using the Advanced Search feature, one can target search results to journal articles available in full text. The Directory of Open Access Journals (www.doaj.org), a source of scientific and scholarly literature, also provides access to journals printed in all languages. This directory is housed at Lund University in Sweden and includes journals in the health and social sciences.

Other sources on the Internet provide either free or partially free access to quality-controlled summaries of systematic reviews. The Campbell Collaboration (http://www.campbellcollaboration.org) provides free access to systematic reviews in the areas of education, social welfare, and crime and justice. Although the abstracts and plain language summaries of Cochrane Collaboration (http://www.cochrane.org) reviews are open to all, access to the full reviews are available only through an institution or individual subscription. OT Search, jointly supported by AOTA and the American Occupational Therapy Foundation (http://www1.aota.org/otsearch/index.asp), offers material at nominal cost and may be valuable if the information is not available elsewhere. OT Search is also a good source if one is interested specifically in focusing on occupational therapy–specific journals or authors.

CHECKING ADDITIONAL SOURCES OF CITATIONS

Although a database search may reveal most citations in the literature, additional techniques should be used to uncover other articles. Examining the reference lists of articles included in a review and the publication lists of important researchers in a given field may reveal important research not picked up by the bibliographic search. Another method of finding relevant articles is hand searching the literature. Each area of research has a journal or journals that are central to the field. By going through the tables of contents of back issues of those journals, one may locate important articles. Authors can identify the journals that provide information about the focused question by searching the Internet using search terms that combine the diagnosis or clinical condition with the term *journal,* by consulting with a research librarian, or by asking experts in the field for suggestions. Journals with electronic access maintain an archive of past issues, simplifying the process of reviewing tables of contents for several years.

KEEPING TRACK OF THE RESULTS

Because search results may be hundreds of pages long, it is best to handle this information electronically as opposed to having a printout of citations and abstracts. Highlighting potentially useful articles and then creating a separate file of these studies can also be helpful. Developing a system to document the output of the search helps authors track articles retrieved. A simple method is to create a citation table with columns for the full citation of an article, research design and level of evidence (described in the next section), and whether it passed the final cut for inclusion or notation of the reason for exclusion. A citation table allows other team members to discuss the choices made for inclusion and exclusion and is subsequently used in writing the methodology section of the systematic review.

Using the Critical Appraisal Process

Once the search is complete, the author or team members review the titles and abstracts of the articles to determine if they should be included, rejected, or reviewed further before making a final decision. The criteria for screening articles specified in the protocol guide their decisions. The full text of the articles that pass this first stage can then be retrieved for critical appraisal.

Two formats can be used to document the information gained from the critical appraisal process—critically appraised papers (CAPs) and evidence tables—and both are extremely helpful at the later stage of writing the systematic review article. A critically appraised paper is an at-a-glance summary of an article written using a structured format, and it can help authors new to the systematic review process get comfortable with the important components of critical appraisal. For more information on writing a CAP, visit the AOTA Evidence-Based Practice Project's Evidence Exchange (http://www.aota.org/Educate/Research.aspx). The following materials can be found there:

> **Occupational therapy and other clinical disciplines use standards of evidence modeled on those developed in evidence-based medicine.**

- CAP worksheet
- CAP guidelines
- *CAP Submission Toolkit*
- *Evidence Exchange CAP Developer Training*
- *Research Statistics 101 for EBP.*

An evidence table is a simple and concise format for organizing abbreviated summaries of the articles. Information on developing evidence tables can be found in the author guidelines for the *American Journal of Occupational Therapy,* which are published yearly (see AOTA, 2012). Both CAPs and evidence tables describe the strength and quality of the evidence in terms of the study's objectives, level of evidence, design, intervention, outcome measures, and results.

OBJECTIVES

The objectives of the study provide the justification for the research and help the review authors determine the value of the research to the focused question.

DESIGN AND LEVELS OF EVIDENCE

Occupational therapy and other clinical disciplines use standards of evidence modeled on those developed in evidence-based medicine. This model standardizes and ranks the value of scientific evidence using the grading system in Table 10.1. This is one example of grading systems that have been developed:

- The highest level of evidence, *Level I,* includes randomized controlled trials, systematic reviews of the literature, and meta-analyses.

TABLE 10.1. Levels of Evidence for Occupational Therapy Outcomes Research

Level of Evidence	Definitions
Level I	Systematic reviews, meta-analyses, randomized controlled trials
Level II	Two groups, nonrandomized studies (e.g., cohort, case–control)
Level III	One group, nonrandomized (e.g., before and after, pretest and posttest)
Level IV	Descriptive studies that include analysis of outcomes (e.g., single-subject design, case series)
Level V	Case reports and expert opinion that include narrative literature reviews and consensus statements

Note. Adapted from "Evidence-Based Medicine: What It Is and What It Isn't," by D. L. Sackett, W. M. Rosenberg, J. A. Muir Gray, R. B. Haynes, & W. S. Richardson, 1996, *British Medical Journal*, *312*, pp. 71–72. Copyright © 1996 by the British Medical Association. Adapted with permission.

Randomized controlled trials compare the outcomes of an intervention group with the outcomes of a control group, and participation in either group is determined randomly. This design is the best available to support the conclusion that the effect (dependent variable) was caused by the treatment (independent variable).

- In *Level II* studies, assignment to a treatment or a control group is not randomized (cohort study).
- *Level III* studies do not use a control group.
- *Level IV* studies are experimental single-case studies with at least some manipulation of the independent variable.
- *Level V* evidence includes narrative reviews, consensus statements, and descriptive case reports in which therapists simply describe what they did and what the outcome was for one or a few persons.

In many systematic reviews, if Level I, II, or III evidence for occupational therapy practice is adequate, then only studies at those levels are used to answer a particular question. If, however, higher-level evidence is lacking and the best evidence provided for occupational therapy specifically is ranked at Levels IV and V, then studies at those levels are included.

Although qualitative research typically is not included in systematic reviews, some reviews include qualitative studies when evidence at higher levels is lacking. Qualitative study designs are rooted in the naturalistic research paradigm in which researcher subjectivity is seen as an essential component of the investigation, not as a source of bias (Guba & Lincoln, 1989; Scheer, Arbesman, & Lieberman, 2008). Mary Law, Lori Letts, and their colleagues in the EBP Working Group at McMaster University in Hamilton, Ontario, developed critical appraisal techniques (Law, 2002; Law & MacDermid, 2007) that articulate the dimensions and technical procedures used in trustworthy qualitative research (Guba & Lincoln, 1989). These techniques address study design, theoretical perspective, study population, data collection, and auditability (i.e., analytic trail, data triangulation, multiple coding, participant validation/member check), and the rigor of a qualitative study and the trustworthiness of findings can be assessed on the basis of the extent to which the study adheres to these techniques.

In addition, information on the analysis of qualitative research can be found at the Web site of the Joanna Briggs Institute, in the section Thematic Analysis Program under Appraise Evidence (http://www.joannabriggs.edu. au/Home). Qualitative methodologists have also developed procedures for aggregating or pooling findings from groups of qualitative studies to produce the results of systematic reviews of the qualitative evidence to contribute to the development of EBP (Holmes & Pearson, 2004; Sandelowski & Barroso, 2007; Sandelowski, Docherty, & Emden, 1997).

PARTICIPANTS

In summarizing information on the participants in the study, the authors consider several questions:

- What were the characteristics of the sample population included in the review (e.g., diagnosis, age, gender)?
- What were the inclusion and exclusion criteria for the study participants?
- How were the participants recruited?
- Was there a specific setting from which the patients were recruited (e.g., inpatient rehabilitation setting)?
- How many participants were in the sample, and what were the intervention and control group conditions?

INTERVENTION

The summary of the study intervention and the control group process, if appropriate, covers the following:

- Intervention and control group conditions
- Frequency of intervention and control treatment
- Duration of intervention and control treatment
- Setting of the intervention and control treatment.

OUTCOME MEASURES

The outcome measures summary describes how performance was measured at baseline and in any follow-up. This summary should address the following:

- What instruments were used to measure outcomes?
- Were the instruments appropriate for the study?
- Were the instruments appropriate for the focused question?
- Were the instruments reliable and valid?
- Was the assessment process blind? That is, was the intervention condition unknown to the evaluator?

RESULTS

The results section provides detailed information on the outcomes of the research study. The results section may include

- Descriptive data on the characteristics of the group(s) included in the study
- Data on performance on assessment measures at baseline
- Data on performance on assessment measures at follow-up(s)
- Comparison of group performance on outcome measures at follow-up (if appropriate, due to study design).

Many studies, especially by non–occupational therapy researchers, contain results that do not pertain to the focused question of the systematic review. The review authors must craft the summary of results using the lens of the focused question.

The results summary also includes methodological strengths and limitations of the research design:

- Was the study sample large enough (adequately powered) to show a difference?
- Was the duration of the intervention long enough to make a difference?
- Was the follow-up period long enough to demonstrate that the intervention made a difference?
- Was the statistical analysis appropriate for the study design and the study purpose?
- Were the conclusions justified?
- If a statistically significant difference was found, do the results have clinical significance? That is, will implementing the intervention make a difference in clinical practice?
- Could any conflicts of interest in carrying out the study have influenced the study outcome and interpretation of results?

Assessments are available for use in rating the quality, strengths, and limitations of an individual intervention study (Downs & Black, 1998; MacDermid, 2004; Moher et al., 1995; Physiotherapy Evidence Database, n.d.). Although some can be used only with randomized or nonrandomized controlled trials, others can also be used for other study designs. These assessments provide a summary of the critical appraisal process of each article included in a systematic review.

Writing the Systematic Review Article

The systematic review article is usually divided into sections on the focused question, background, methodology, results, and discussion. The focused question, background, and methodology sections are descriptive and straightforward; this section focuses on the results and discussion sections.

Determining themes or categories of findings can help authors structure the results section. For narrowly focused questions, one or two themes may suffice, but broader questions may involve several themes. The terminology of the *Occupational Therapy Practice Framework: Domain and Process* (AOTA, 2008) can be used to organize expansive topics into areas of occupation, performance skills and performance patterns, environment and context, client factors, and activity demands and subthemes within these topic areas. Within each theme and subtheme, the evidence is organized by level of evidence. A review with many studies can present evidence at each level separately. Reviews with fewer studies can group studies with higher levels of evidence (e.g., I, II, and III) together in one section and studies with lower levels in another. Grading systems, such as one developed by the U.S. Preventive Services Task Force (http://www.uspreventiveservicestaskforce.org/uspstf/grades.htm), are useful for determining the strength of the evidence in a given theme.

For systematic reviews in which there is clinical homogeneity of results within the themes, it may be possible to pool the results and conduct a meta-analysis of the results (Moher, Jadad, & Klassen, 1998; Palisano, 2008; Wright et al., 2007). Individual studies included in a meta-analysis need to have used reliable and valid measures for assessment, with results reported using inferential statistics (e.g., t test, analysis of variance), and the results are reported using odds ratios and effect sizes. The discussion section describes the implications of the findings for clinical practice, education, research, and policy as appropriate. At this point in the research and writing process, the authors stretch themselves creatively and ask, What are the possibilities for this evidence? Collaboration ensures that the discussion section addresses all possibilities; team members and other reviewers within and outside occupational therapy may suggest additional ideas about the implications of the results of the systematic review.

The limitations of the studies included in the systematic review can be presented in either the results or the discussion section. The summaries of study limitations written during the critical appraisal of each article contribute to the discussion of the overall limitations of the entire review. Common limitations encountered in studies include small sample size, lack of a control group or randomization, limited follow-up period, inadequate description of the intervention and control group conditions, absence of data on the reliability and validity of assessment measures, and failure to use an attention placebo for the comparison group.

Submitting the Article for Publication

Both peer-reviewed and non-peer-reviewed journals publish systematic review articles. Appropriate peer-reviewed journals may include occupational therapy and rehabilitation journals, as well as some specialty journals that focus on an individual diagnosis or clinical condition. Examples of occupational therapy journals include the following:

- *American Journal of Occupational Therapy*
- *Australian Occupational Therapy Journal*
- *British Journal of Occupational Therapy*
- *Canadian Journal of Occupational Therapy*
- *Journal of Occupational Therapy, Schools, and Early Intervention*
- *Occupational Therapy in Health Care*
- *Occupational Therapy International.*

Examples of rehabilitation journals include the following:

- *American Journal of Physical Medicine and Rehabilitation*
- *Archives of Physical Medicine and Rehabilitation*
- *Clinical Rehabilitation*
- *Journal of NeuroEngineering and Rehabilitation*
- *Journal of Rehabilitation Medicine*
- *Journal of Rehabilitation Research and Development*
- *The Open Rehabilitation Journal.*

Peer-reviewed journals have specific submission criteria, and although the focus may be on clinical practice, they place a strong emphasis on research and academics.

For authors interested in reaching a clinically based audience, non-peer-reviewed publications such as *OT Practice* and the AOTA Special Interest Section newsletters have wide audiences that are eager to read the results of well-conducted systematic reviews. Non-peer-reviewed publications tend to place emphasis on implications for practice.

Choosing a journal to submit to will depend on the intended audience. Authors also need to keep in mind that an article should be submitted to only one journal at a time. The article submitted must carefully follow the author guidelines and reference format for the selected journal. In addition, the systematic review components included should be tailored to the journal's emphasis (e.g., underlying research and theory, implications for practice). Finally, the search terms and databases can be summarized in a table format and included in the manuscript.

> **Authors also need to keep in mind that an article should be submitted to only one journal at a time.**

Writing Systematic Reviews

Systematic reviews provide crucial information to occupational therapy practitioners. Research findings, combined with individual clinical expertise, enable practitioners to provide interventions to their clients that are both up to date and scientifically based.

REFERENCES

American Occupational Therapy Association. (2008). Occupational therapy practice framework: Domain and process (2nd ed.). *American Journal of Occupational Therapy, 62,* 625–683. doi:10.5014/ajot.62.6.625

American Occupational Therapy Association. (2012). Guidelines for contributors. Retrieved November 20, 2012, from http://www.aota.org/DocumentVault/AJOT/Guidelines-Tables.aspx

American Occupational Therapy Association. (n.d.). *Evidence-based practice and research.* Retrieved August 6, 2011, from http://www.aota.org/Practitioners/PracticeAreas/Work/Evidence.aspx

Collins, J. A., & Fauser, B. C. (2005). Balancing the strengths of systematic and narrative reviews. *Human Reproduction Update, 11,* 103–104.

Cook, D. J., Sackett, D. L., & Spitzer, W. O. (1995). Methodologic guidelines for systematic reviews of randomized control trials in health care from the Potsdam Consultation on Meta-Analysis. *Journal of Clinical Epidemiology, 48,* 167–171.

Downs, S. H., & Black, N. (1998). The feasibility of creating a checklist for the assessment of the methodological quality both of randomised and non-randomised studies of health care interventions. *Journal of Epidemiology and Community Health, 52,* 377–384.

Edward G. Miner Library, University of Rochester Medical Center. (n.d.). *Evidence-based filters for Ovid CINAHL.* Retrieved October 14, 2012, from www.urmc.rochester.edu/hslt/miner/digital_library/tip_sheets/cinahl_eb_filters.pdf

Guba, E. G., & Lincoln, Y. S. (1989). Judging the quality of fourth generation evaluation. In *Fourth generation evaluation* (pp. 228–251). Thousand Oaks, CA: Sage.

Holm, M. B. (2000). Our mandate for the new millennium: Evidence-based practice (Eleanor Clarke Slagle Lecture). *American Journal of Occupational Therapy, 54,* 575–585. doi:10.5014/ajot.54.6.575

Holmes, C., & Pearson, A. (2004). The metasynthesis of qualitative research findings in evidence-based health care. *Joanna Briggs Institute Reports, 2*(4), 33–44.

Institute of Medicine. (2008). *Knowing what works in health care: A roadmap for the nation.* Washington, DC: National Academies Press.

Law, M. (2002). *Evidence-based rehabilitation: A guide to practice.* Thorofare, NJ: Slack.

Law, M., & Baum, C. (1998). Evidence-based occupational therapy. *Canadian Journal of Occupational Therapy, 65,* 131–135.

Law, M., & MacDermid, J. (2007). *Evidence-based rehabilitation: A guide to practice* (2nd ed.). Thorofare, NJ: Slack.

Lin, S. H., Murphy, S. L., & Robinson, J. C. (2010). The issue is—Facilitating evidence-based practice. *American Journal of Occupational Therapy, 64,* 164–171. doi:10.5014/ajot.64.1.164

MacDermid, J. C. (2004). An introduction to evidence-based practice for hand therapists. *Journal of Hand Therapy, 17,* 108–117.

Moher, D., Jadad, A. R., & Klassen, T. P. (1998). Guides for reading and interpreting systematic reviews III. How did the authors synthesize the data and make their conclusions? *Archives of Pediatrics & Adolescent Medicine, 152,* 915–920.

Moher, D., Jadad, A. R., Nichol, G., Penman, M., Tugwell, P., & Walsh, S. (1995). Assessing the quality of randomized controlled trials: An annotated bibliography of scales and checklists. *Controlled Clinical Trials, 16,* 62–73.

Murphy, S. L., Robinson, J. C., & Lin, S. H. (2009). Conducting systematic reviews to inform occupational therapy practice. *American Journal of Occupational Therapy, 63,* 363–368. doi:10.5014/ajot.63.3.363

National Institutes of Health. (2012). *National Institutes of Health public access policy.* Retrieved October 14, 2012, from http://publicaccess.nih.gov/

Palisano, R. J. (2008). Submitting a systematic review. *Physical & Occupational Therapy in Pediatrics, 28,* 209–213. doi:10.1080/01942630802031784

Physiotherapy Evidence Database. (n.d.). *PEDro scale (partitioned): Rating sheet.* Retrieved August 7, 2011, from http://www.otseeker.com/PDF/PEDroscale partitionedratingsheet.pdf

Sackett, D. L., Rosenberg, W. M., Muir Gray, J. A., Haynes, R. B., & Richardson, W. S. (1996). Evidence-based medicine: What it is and what it isn't. *British Medical Journal, 312,* 71–72.

Sandelowski, M., & Barroso, J. (2007). *Handbook for synthesizing qualitative research.* New York: Springer.

Sandelowski, M., Docherty, S., & Emden, C. (1997). Qualitative meta-synthesis: Issues and techniques. *Research in Nursing and Health, 20,* 365–371.

Scheer, J., Arbesman, M., & Lieberman, D. (2008). Using findings from qualitative studies as evidence to inform practice: An update. *OT Practice, 13*(10), 15–18.

Suber, P. (2004). *Open access overview.* Retrieved August 6, 2011, from http://www.earlham.edu/~peters/fos/overview.htm

Tickle-Degnen, L. (1999). Evidence-based Practice Forum—Organizing, evaluating, and using evidence in occupational therapy practice. *American Journal of Occupational Therapy, 53,* 537–539.

Wright, R. W., Brand, R. A., Dunn, W., & Spindler, K. P. (2007). How to write a systematic review. *Clinical Orthopaedics and Related Research, 455,* 23–29.

11

An Introduction to Grant Writing

LEONARD G. TRUJILLO, PhD, OTR/L

There is grant money available for just about anything if you know where to look and how to write the proposal.

—CYNTHIA KNOWLES (2002, p. 1)

A strong characteristic of occupational therapists is their desire to improve the lives of the clients and populations they serve. Occupational therapists are among the most inventive and creative of individuals, but creativity alone is not sufficient to make dreams a reality. Through projects funded by grants, occupational therapists can transition from inventive individuals into a profession of respected innovators in research and practice and in so doing enact the *Centennial Vision* of occupational therapy as "a powerful, widely recognized, science-driven, and evidence-based profession with a globally connected and diverse workforce meeting society's occupational needs" (American Occupational Therapy Association, 2007, p. 613).

As with most worthwhile ventures in life, grant-funded projects often begin with a notion or an idea that someone has and wants to implement. Say you have a new concept, idea, treatment intervention, or program, but to put it into practice you must find funding. By applying for a grant, you may be able to obtain this funding from a government source or group of individuals who wish to make a difference in society. This chapter discusses sources of grant funding, requests for proposals (RFPs), the basics of and tips for writing a grant proposal (for more in-depth discussion, consult the resources in the "Recommended Reading" list), and some of the myths people encounter about grant writing. In addition, Appendix 11.A contains a glossary of grant-related terms; please consult the appendix if terms in this chapter are unfamiliar to you.

Sources of Grant Funding

Before spending time diving into the grant proposal itself, you should identify and investigate potential funding or grantors (Dahlen, 2001). If possible, read about studies or grants each funder has already funded. Obviously, you don't want to repeat what someone else has done, but it helps to know what a grantor has funded in the past. Go to the funder's Web site, and click on the tab or button that says "About Us."

Government grants are funded to address current needs and priorities that are of public interest. Recent emphases include innovative technologies and development in such areas as agriculture, business and commerce, community development, energy, housing, and education, as well as newer opportunities through the American Recovery and Reinvestment Act of 2009. Grants.gov, a central storehouse for information on federal agencies that award grants, posts information about grants, topic areas, and specific grants that are open for submission of proposals.

The federal government funds several categories of grants, including research, demonstration, project, block, and formula grants. The categories indicate the type of grant and expected outcome. For example, research grants fund investigation into scientific, quantifiable questions and have measurable outcomes. Research grant programs seek to discover facts, challenge or revise theories, and apply new theories (U.S. Department of Agriculture, Rural Information Center, 2009). Demonstration or block grants are often used to provide or enhance the delivery of occupational therapy services to a given population.

Private funding sources, such as foundations, corporations, volunteer agencies, and community groups, fund projects in areas of particular interest (U.S. Department of Agriculture, Rural Information Center, 2009).

Finding sources for private funding can be challenging. Watch for announcements sent to your work setting; settings with a grants office have staff who are aware of potential funding sources. Consider possibilities in the local community, such as foundations linked to medical centers and corporations. Searching on the Internet using key words describing your topics of interest and *funding opportunities* may turn up useful Web sites; for example, the Social Psychology Network (www.socialpsychology.org/funding.htm) provides links to major grantmaking foundations.

It is your responsibility to investigate and match your project to the interests of the foundation. Again, grantors' Web sites have a wealth of information. Reading grant proposals previously submitted to a grantor provides insight into not only the types of projects they have been willing to fund (Hoibrook, 2001) but also the writing styles and readability of successful proposals. Some Web sites post answers to questions that others have had about, for example, the submission process, formatting, and what is and isn't acceptable. If past proposals aren't available on the Web site or to request clarification of submission requirements and expectations, contact the organization using the contact information provided on the Web site.

Requests for Proposals

Once you have selected a potential funding source and identified a specific grant announcement, read the request for proposals once, and then read it again . . . and again. Several readings of an RFP are necessary for a thorough understanding of what the grantor requires in a proposal. RFPs have sections designated by letters that are generally the same across RFPs (e.g., Section B refers to pricing, Section C to scope of work, Section K to representations and certifications, Section L to instructions for bidders, Section M to bid evaluation criteria). Descriptions of information critical to include in your submission may be scattered among many different sections of an RFP (Grants.gov, 2010; Office of Extramural Research, National Institutes of Health [NIH], 2011; Recovery.gov, 2010).

After familiarizing yourself with the RFP and the funder's expectations, you may still have questions. Don't be intimidated about requesting information and assistance from the funder; submitting your inquiries to the funder helps ensure your proposal will be in the best position possible for success. Submit questions in writing to the contracting officer identified in the RFP. Some RFPs specify a date by which questions are due; questions sent after the due date may not be considered. Some grantors' Web sites post questions sent in by others who are considering submitting a proposal along with the grantor responses. Also, monitor the Web site for amendments that describe significant changes to the RFP (Grants.gov, 2010; Office of Extramural Research, NIH, 2011; Recovery.com, 2010).

Each funding agency has its own rules and guidelines for submission of proposals; basic components of these guidelines are discussed later in this chapter. Grant reviewers often comment that the first round of elimination weeds out those who have submitted their proposal without following the directions. Once you have decided to submit a proposal, obtain the grantor's submission guidelines. Allowing yourself sufficient time to follow the grantor's rules for submission will ensure that your valued concept will be considered (Egan, 2006).

Just as important as understanding and following the rules of the grantor is abiding by your own institution's internal rules for submitting grant proposals. The structured process outlined in institutional rules is important to layer on top of the grantor's guidelines for submission. Thus, giving sufficient time for internal review before submitting your grant proposal is an additional consideration you must build into your timeline.

Writing the Grant Proposal

Grant proposals can be as simple as a single-page outline of a proposed implementation submitted by a single primary investigator or as complicated as a multiple-page, multiagency project with coinvestigators at every research site. Some grant applicants initiate their first grant request in the form of writing a letter to a vendor and asking for a discount to test a new equipment design or treatment protocol. They then build on that experience,

> Grant proposals can be as simple as a single-page outline of a proposed implementation submitted by a single primary investigator or as complicated as a multiple-page, multiagency project with coinvestigators at every research site.

progressing through increasingly complex proposals. The basic concepts of submission at any level are similar: You have a concept that needs financial support, so you outline in writing what the idea is, describe what is needed to make it successful, and justify how you will know that it was completed successfully. Everything else in a grant proposal adds detail to these basic elements.

The Office of Extramural Research at NIH (2011) outlined the following five areas that are critical in proposal development:

1. *Significance:* Your proposal must convince reviewers that your project addresses an important or critical problem you have identified. You should speak specifically to what the grantor identifies as its funding purpose; the focus is not on how important the grant will be for your study or work, but rather on how your work is of significance to the grantor's needs or desires. Reviewers may also want to know how your project will improve the knowledge base and understanding of the problem you are addressing and generate new concepts to improve outcomes.

2. *Investigators:* The reviewers will examine the description of the primary investigator or project officer, including his or her qualifications and background and any track record of completed grant-funded projects. In essence, you are interviewing for a position, and the reviewers will try to determine if you are the right one for the job. Differentiation of degrees and past experience can be critical; if you have a specialty certification in your area of expertise, be sure to note it.

3. *Innovation:* Many grantors are looking for new and innovative approaches to addressing the problem as defined. Novelty and creativity are essential to your description of your approach and can help you overcome reviewer hesitancy. Many recent grants that have federal government funding are in the general category of innovation and technology. This is where occupational therapists can excel in their description of what they do: Describe how your proposal will make a difference in people's lives.

4. *Approach:* Reviewers will look for a clear description of your methodology and plan for analyzing the data you collect. Include a description of the limitations of your design, and describe how you will address these limitations. Be sure to describe the populations to be affected by your work, including minority populations.

5. *Environment:* Your proposal must describe the characteristics of the environment in which you are working, including whether it is accepting of or antagonistic toward your project. Also describe the extent of institutional support you can count on; such support adds to the probability of success in the eyes of reviewers. Exploring the possibilities within your community takes extra effort, and finding and contacting the right people in your community is fundamental, particularly if you are working with military or government agencies. Establishing memorandums of understanding and submitting them with the grant proposal as an attachment of support will strengthen your proposal.

BASIC COMPONENTS

Many grant proposal processes have a preproposal process in which you submit a preliminary, less detailed view of your proposal for the funder to review. If it makes it through this review, you are asked to submit a more comprehensive and detailed write-up for final review.

Although there is some variation, most grantors require the following components:

- *Project title:* The ideal title both catches attention and briefly describes the project being proposed (Non-profit Guides, 2013). Your title should be descriptive, like a very short abstract; avoid cute or catchy titles.
- *Applicant information:* Applicant information includes who you are, the organization you represent, and essential personal background information. Identify all people who are contributing to the work that is being proposed, and outline who will be responsible for what (Non-profit Guides, 2013). Gathering applicant information can be time-consuming, so everyone must have their biographical information, including degrees and certifications, up to date and ready for submission.
- *Project summary:* The summary is a statement of what the project is and will do. Describe clearly and concisely how you intend to achieve the goals in sufficient detail that reviewers clearly understand what your intentions are and how what you are proposing is doable (Non-profit Guides, 2013). Often grantors place a restriction on the space to be used for the project summary (e.g., 250 words).
- *Statement of need:* This statement clearly describes the need your project is going to meet. Do not assume the reviewers know the problems that exist; reviewers may not be part of the grantor organization or

understand or see the world as you do. What value will your project contribute toward? What need will it help resolve? Who will directly benefit from the project, and how will you measure the outcomes you are expecting (Non-profit Guides, 2013)?

- *Program objectives:* Your objectives clearly state what you expect to accomplish. Give expected milestones and time frames and planned methods for reporting the outcomes. Be explicit about how your project will achieve the stated objectives and how you will evaluate the effectiveness of the project (Non-profit Guides, 2013).

- *Budget outline:* This section provides a justification of expenses and identifies where the grantor's money is to be spent (e.g., personnel, equipment, rent; Nonprofit Guides, 2013). Provide a list of specific items you need, explaining why each expenditure is important. Many grantors will not allow you to spend money differently than specified in your proposal, so realistic expense projections are essential to a successful project. In addition, make sure your budget expenses fall within the spending regulations of your institution. For example, if you are in a university setting that prohibits paying for student travel, obtaining grant money for that expense does not give you the authority to spend it in that fashion. All funding is subject to the regulations and rules of your work setting.

- *Summary:* The summary, like an abstract, provides an overview of your proposal that is concise and synthesizes your intent. Use terms that are descriptive of what you are doing (e.g., *service, research*). Tout the uniqueness of the proposal, and assure readers that you have everything in place to accomplish the proposal once you have financial support (Non-profit Guides, 2013). In addition, review your qualifications to carry out your project.

Grantors (especially the federal government) will evaluate your proposal on the basis only of the specific information contained within it; you should assume that they are completely unaware of your organization's capabilities, staff, and past projects. You must describe everything thoroughly in accordance with RFP instructions.

SCHEDULE

Create a schedule for submitting your grant proposal, and make an effort to stick with it. Identify the deadline date and work backward, assigning time frames and deadlines to get each of the submission requirements done. If you are working with others, distribute the schedule to all members of your team.

Rather than putting the easier requirements off until the last minute (e.g., bio sketches of the principal investigator and collaborators), get them done early so you begin to feel a sense of momentum. If a background statement is required, get started early on doing the literature review and gathering information. You might want to make a separate schedule for preparation of the budget.

Make sure you leave plenty of time for copying, binding, and delivering the proposal. Remember, Murphy's Law will strike, and the copier can sense that an important document is being copied, so it's sure to break, jam, or smudge. Have a backup plan that includes having extra paper and toner on hand or sending the proposal out to be copied. For grantors that have changed to an electronic review process, you may need to invest in software that transforms your documents into an acceptable format. Be sure you know what the submission process is within your institution; most institutions have a single submission portal for federal grant submissions. Again, knowing what the internal process is well ahead of time can make or break the successful submission of your proposal.

TIPS FOR PROPOSAL PREPARATION

This section provides tips for keeping things organized as you develop the different sections and elements of your submission.

Constructing an Outline

Requests for grant proposals often contain an outline or list of requirements for submission. Download the RFP, and use that file to construct your proposal outline.

- Save one version with the basic outline, and save another version as a spreadsheet or table listing the status of each section and associated deadlines to annotate regularly.
- If you're writing the proposal as part of a team, use the annotated version to identify who is writing each section, and indicate the estimated number of pages they will write.
- Put any special or specific requirements and instructions at the top of the list so you do not forget them. These instructions might include proposal due date and time, number of copies, page limits, font size, page margins, and packaging and delivery instructions (Grants.gov, 2010; Office of Extramural Research, NIH, 2011; Recovery.gov, 2010).
- Electronically scan any letters of support and other supporting documents, and save them in pdf format.

Managing Development of the Sections

As we have seen, grant proposals are made up of different sections. You can keep section drafts organized either electronically or by printing the documents and placing then in a binder as they are completed.

- Keep section drafts in a folder or binder with a divider between each section to allow easy access so you can see what has been completed and what is in need of work. Find a method that works for you to track levels of completeness, and use highlighting or sticky notes to mark important pages or paragraphs so you can find them quickly. Label electronic files with the section, date, and status of the document; careful labeling of files can help you keep track of updates and edits along the way.
- Follow all instructions in the Evaluation Section of the RFP. Study the proposal evaluation criteria and the points allocated to each section and subsection of the proposal, as well as the points that are allocated to cost. This information will tell you what to emphasize and where to concentrate your efforts in preparing your proposal.
- Review your work to ensure that you have answered the fundamental questions of who, what, when, where, how, and why (Grants.gov, 2010; Office of Extramural Research, NIH, 2011; Recovery.gov, 2010).
- In the Personnel Section, you may be required to include narrative information on the experience and skills of the team members you are proposing for the project or their résumés. Maintain short bios of each team member, and early in the process, specify their roles in the work to be done should funding be provided (Grants.gov, 2010; Office of Extramural Research, NIH, 2011; Recovery.gov, 2010).
- Use tables, charts, and graphics to summarize information and break up your narrative. Many reviewers appreciate a chart or graphic depiction of how the project is going to be conducted (Grants.gov, 2010; Office of Extramural Research, NIH, 2011; Recovery.gov, 2010).

Developing a Sound Budget

Two common pitfalls in establishing a budget for grant proposals are underestimating costs and adding costs to meet the anticipated amount of the grant. The following steps can maximize the accuracy of your budget:

- Budgeting and planning are best accomplished using a spreadsheet to list the items and keep a running cost calculation. Be sure to include benefits and other nonsalary costs in personnel costing. Prepare a spreadsheet template or checklist of items to be included in your budget.

- Make sure your budget is consistent with what you are proposing to do or provide. Often the RFP specifies that you include a Cost Justifications sheet following the budget items on which you write a short justification for each item (Grants.gov, 2010; Office of Extramural Research, NIH, 2011; Recovery.gov, 2010).

- Estimates are often part of the challenge. Use your personal experience in managing budgets, or ask for assistance in putting together realistic cost estimates. A well-developed budget will indicate to funders your readiness to be a player in the grant arena.

- Check and recheck your numbers and formulas. Proofreading a print copy or having the software read the numbers back to you is a good way to check the accuracy of budgeted allocations (Grants.gov, 2010; Office of Extramural Research, NIH, 2011; Recovery.gov, 2010).

- Make sure that your budget can be easily read. Don't use a font that is too small.

FINAL QUALITY CHECK

One additional method of critiquing your work before submitting it is to ask a trusted colleague to review it using highly critical criteria. A primary source of insightful information on developing and submitting grant proposals is found on the NIH Web site (Office of Extramural Research, NIH, 2011). Applying NIH's peer review criteria to your own grant submission will enhance your submission, regardless of whom you are submitting to.

Once you have completed the proposal, check it in its entirety for the following: spelling; page numbering; section and subsection numbering or lettering; consistency in appearance of headings, subheadings, and font types and sizes; and consistency in technical language. Make sure you have filled in and signed all the forms the RFP requires you to return with your submission. Before and after copying your technical and cost proposals, check to see that each copy contains all pages and that they are in the proper order.

Myths About Grant Writing

You may have heard myths about grant writing that have discouraged you from giving it a try. One such myth is that if you are a first-time grant applicant, you will be turned down (Henson, 2003). This myth comes true only if you fail to do the demanding work that is associated with successful grant writing. So many variables affect selection, and inexperience in grant writing is but one. Grant writing is a craft and a skill that, like any other, needs to be developed. Your first attempts may be turned down, but often you will receive valuable feedback you can use to make changes that will result in a successful future submission. Many grant opportunities go through rotation cycles that will allow you to resubmit, possibly within the same year.

> **Probably the most widespread of all myths is that only the big players get grants and that smaller projects are at a disadvantage . . . . Although there is some validity to this myth, smaller, startup grants are available. Selecting RFPs consistent with your resources is part of a successful grant-writing effort.**

Another myth often voiced is that the only way to get a grant is to have a successful grant writer do the work for you. Although an experienced writer can improve your chances, your ability to successfully obtain a grant depends mostly on your ability to persuade grantors of the merits of your program (Henson, 2003).

Probably the most widespread of all myths is that only the big players get grants and that smaller projects are at a disadvantage (Henson, 2003). Although there is some validity to this myth, smaller, startup grants are available. Selecting RFPs consistent with your resources is part of a successful grant-writing effort.

Writing Your Grant

Occupational therapists need not be limited by the resources currently available in their workplaces. Grants provide many opportunities for occupational therapists to make the shift from clinical practitioner to grant writer and research or practice innovator. A grant proposal describes an activity you intend to carry out and the measureable outcomes you expect following implementation. Your proposal must identify clear objectives for what you intend to do. Your process and measureable outcomes must stand out and clearly be seen as doable. You must translate your passion for your project into clearly stated processes, means of implementation, measurement techniques, and outcomes. In short, you must communicate what you intend to do, how you will measure it, and how you know that what you are doing will have a viable and valued outcome.

REFERENCES

American Occupational Therapy Association. (2007). *Centennial Vision* and executive summary. *American Journal of Occupational Therapy, 61,* 613–614.

American Recovery and Reinvestment Act of 2009, Pub. L. 111–5, 123 Stat. 115, 516.

Browning, B. A. (2009). *Grant writing for dummies* (3rd ed.). Hoboken, NJ: Wiley.

Center for Energy Workforce Development. (n.d.). *ABCs of grant writing.* Washington, DC: Author. Retrieved from http://www.cewd.org/toolkits/grants/abcs_of_grantwriting.pdf

Dahlen, R. (2001). Fundamentals of grant writing: Lessons learned from the process. *Nurse Education, 26*(2), 54–56.

Doll, J. D. (2010). *Program development and grant writing in occupational therapy: Making the connection.* Sudbury, MA: Jones & Bartlett.

Egan, K. (2006). *Top 10 grant writing mistakes.* Retrieved October 29, 2010, from http://www.nsls.info/articles/detail.aspx?articleID=49

Grants.gov. (2010). *Tips and resources from grantors.* Retrieved October 15, 2010, from http://www.grants.gov/applicants/tips_resources_from_grantors.jsp

Henson, K. T. (2003). Debunking some myths about grant writing. *Chronicle of Higher Education.* Retrieved October 5, 2011, from http://chronicle.com/article/Debunking-Some-Myths-About/45256/

Hoibrook, B. (2001). Searching for grants. *Book Report, 19*(4), 51–52.

Knowles, C. (2002). *The first-time grantwriter's guide to success.* Thousand Oaks, CA: Corwin Press.

Non-profit Guides. (2013). *Grant writing tools for nonprofit organizations.* Retrieved April 17, 2013, from http://www.npguides.org

Office of Extramural Research, National Institutes of Health. (2011). *Grant writing tips sheets.* Retrieved October 5, 2011, from http://grants1.nih.gov/grants/grant_tips.htm

Recovery.gov. (2010). *Recovery.* Retrieved October 5, 2011, from http://www.recovery.gov/Pages/default.aspx

U.S. Department of Agriculture, Rural Information Center. (2009). *A guide to funding resources.* Retrieved October 10, 2011, from http://www.nal.usda.gov/ric/ricpubs/fundguide.html

RECOMMENDED READING

Anderson, C. (2003). Write a grant today. *Library Media Connection, 21*(4), 44.

Beitz, J. M., & Bliss, D. Z. (2005). Preparing a successful grant proposal: Part 1. Developing research aims and the significance of the project. *Journal of Wound, Ostomy and Continence Nursing, 32,* 16–18.

Berg, K. M., Gill, T. M., Brown, A. F., Zerzan, J., Elmore, J. G., & Wilson, I. B. (2007). Demystifying the NIH grant application process. *Journal of General Internal Medicine, 22,* 1587–1595.

Burke, M. A. (2002). *Simplified grantwriting.* Thousand Oaks, CA: Corwin Press.

Chambless, D. L. (2003). Hints for writing a NIMH grant. *Behavior Therapist, 26,* 258–261.

Coley, S. M., & Scheinberg, C. A. (2008). *Proposal writing: Effective grantsmanship.* Thousand Oaks, CA: Sage.

Engelfried, S., & Reynolds, A. (2002). Sponsorship 101: How partnerships can expand summer reading. *American Libraries, 33*(2), 49–50.

Fazio, L. S. (2009). *Developing occupation-centered programs for the community.* Upper Saddle River, NJ: Pearson/Prentice Hall.

Gerin, W. (2006). *Writing the NIH grant proposal: A step-by-step guide.* Thousand Oaks, CA: Sage.

Maxwell, J. D. (2005). Money, money, money: Taking the pain out of grant writing. *Teacher Librarian, 32*(3), 16.

Ogden, T., & Goldberg, I. (2002). *Research proposals: A guide to success* (3rd ed.). San Diego, CA: Academic Press.

Reif-Lehrer, L. (2005). *Grant application writer's handbook.* Sudbury, MA: Jones & Bartlett.

Russell, S., & Morrison, D. (2002). *The grant application writer's workbook.* Los Olivos, CA: Grant Writers' Seminars and Workshops.

Sonis, J. H., Triffleman, E., King, L., & King, D. (2009). How to write an NIH R13 conference grant application. *Academic Psychiatry, 33,* 256–260.

U.S. Army. (2009). *Program announcement: Department of Defense Congressionally Directed Medical Research Programs psychological health/traumatic brain injury research program concept award.* Retrieved October 5, 2011, from http://cdmrp.army.mil/funding/pa/09phtbirpiira_pa.pdf

Yang, O. (2005). *Guide to effective grant writing: How to write an effective NIH grant application.* New York: Springer.

Appendix 11.A. Glossary of Grant-Related Terms

block grant—Funding awarded by the federal government to state or local governments for a variety of purposes (e.g., to provide services).

budget justification—List of anticipated expenditures in implementing the project and the rationale for including each item (Doll, 2010, p. 244).

building or renovation funds—Money to build or renovate a facility (Browning, 2009, p. 12; Center for Energy Workforce Development [CEWD], n.d.). Funding often ceases once the project is complete, and the grantee must take over the expenses of operating the facility.

capital support—Money for equipment, buildings, construction, and endowments (Browning, 2009, p. 13); often a one-time grant for items that have a life expectancy of more than 5 years.

cash match—Percentage of the grant's budget that the applying organization must match (Doll, 2010, p. 114).

Catalog of Federal Domestic Assistance (CFDA)—Listing of all federal programs available to government and private entities that provide assistance or benefits to the U.S. public; a CFDA number is assigned to every RFP listed on Grants.gov (Doll, 2010, p. 114).

challenge monies—Grant is approved only if the grantee is able to raise additional money from other sources. For example, the grantor may award a grant of $15,000 if the grantee can raise (or use from existing resources) an additional $5,000 for the specified project.

coinvestigator—Team member listed in the grant proposal who helps implement the program and achieve the grant's goals and objectives (Doll, 2010, p. 114).

collaborative grant—Grant that involves a team approach with multiple investigators who each has a specific assigned role in the program's implementation (Doll, 2010, p. 114).

community foundation—Public foundation that supports a local community and accepts donations to support its programs (Doll, 2010, p. 114).

conference or seminar grant—Money to cover the cost of attending, planning, and/or hosting conferences and seminars; many government conference or seminar grants require the publication of findings (Browning, 2009, p. 13).

consultative grant model—Grant that includes a single principal investigator with coinvestigators, as well as experts who act as consultants and provide feedback on the program as it is implemented (Doll, 2010, p. 114).

consulting grant—Grant to pay for the expertise of a consultant or consulting firm, most often on a one-time or short-term basis, to provide input vital to the success of the grant project (Browning, 2009, p. 13).

continuing support or continuation grant—Grant providing additional funds for the same project (many grantors fund a grantee only once; Browning, 2009, p. 13).

cooperative grant model—Grant that includes more than one principal investigator or that is submitted by more than one institution (Doll, 2010, p. 114).

corporate foundation—Foundation that receives a portion of a corporation's profits to use for philanthropic purposes (Doll, 2010, p. 114).

Data Universal Numbering System (DUNS)—Worldwide system that assigns a unique numeric identifier to business entities; organizations apply for a DUNS number through the federal government (CEWD, n.d.).

deliverables—Services or goods the grantee plans to deliver following a grant award (CEWD, n.d.).

demonstration grant—Grant that funds a study of the feasibility of a new program (Doll, 2010, p. 114).

direct costs—Items in the budget that can be identified specifically with a sponsored project or that can be directly assigned to the project relatively easily and accurately (Doll, 2010, p. 244).

educational grant—Grant that funds implementation of an educational program focused on a specific topic (Doll, 2010, p. 114).

fellowship—(a) Funding for a special project completed by an individual for an organization (Doll, 2010, p. 114); (b) money used to support a graduate or postgraduate student in a specific field (Browning, 2009, p. 13).

financial proposal—Document outlining the costs of providing the needed services or goods; typically separate from budget costs and justifications.

foundation—Private not-for-profit agency with funds to support community programs (Doll, 2010, p. 114).

funding cycle—Timeline of activities in the grant process (e.g., request for proposals, submission, review).

general or operating expenses—Money used for everyday expenses to run an organization, such as salaries, equipment, utilities, travel, and consultants.

goal—Overall purpose of a proposed program (Doll, 2010, p. 244).

grant narrative—The section of the grant proposal that includes the goals, objectives, activities, proposed outcomes, background, needs or problem statement, literature review, theoretical foundation, methodology or implementation plan, timeline, and dissemination plan (Doll, 2010, p. 244).

grant proposal—Application to a government or private entity that describes a project, estimates its costs, and requests monetary assistance; this document often serves as the blueprint for the project (Doll, 2010, p. 244).

grant review—Process in which a peer review panel organized by the funding agency reviews and ranks a submitted grant proposal.

grantee—Person, program, or project receiving grant money (Doll, 2010, p. 114).

grantor—Agency that provides grant money (Doll, 2010, p. 114).

implementation plan—Description of the who, what, where, when, and how of project implementation (Doll, 2010, p. 244).

indirect costs—Expenses not associated readily and specifically with a sponsored project that are incurred for common or joint objectives with other organizational activity (e.g., overhead costs; Doll, 2010, p. 244).

individual grant model—Grant that includes a single principal investigator; the traditional model for research or educational grants (Doll, 2010, p. 114).

matching funds—Funds awarded only if additional funding equal to (or greater than) the grant amount is raised from internal sources, another grant, or donations.

objectives—Proposed program outcomes that will be measured in the evaluation plan (Doll, 2010, p. 244).

outcomes—Results the program proposes to achieve through implementation (Doll, 2010, p. 244).

peer review panel—Anonymous team of people who review grant proposals and select programs to receive funding (Doll, 2010, p. 114).

planning grant—Grant that provides funding for planning a program (Doll, 2010, p. 114).

principal investigator (PI)—Person in charge of the grant program, including development and submission of the grant (Doll, 2010, p. 114). Should the grant be awarded, this person is responsible for overseeing the successful completion of the grant work.

problem statement or needs statement—Description of the problem or need the grant project seeks to address (Doll, 2010, p. 244).

program officer—Main contact for the grant program who is available to answer questions about requests for proposals and program requirements (Doll, 2010, p. 114).

proposing agent—Principal investigator and his or her supporting institution.

request for proposal (RFP)—Public announcement of a funding opportunity; often outlines the application requirements, dates for submission, program requirements, and potential funding amounts and provides contact information for more information.

research grant—Grant that funds projects to address a defined research question (Doll, 2010, p. 115).

subcontract grant model—Grant for which one institution acts as the primary investigator with funding subcontracted to another institution to carry out certain aspects of the project (Doll, 2010, p. 115).

training grant—Grant focused on developing and implementing a specific type of training program (Doll, 2010, p. 115).

12

Writing About Unique Clinical Practice and Innovative Services

WINIFRED SCHULTZ-KROHN, PhD, OTR/L, BCP, SWC, FAOTA

If occupational therapists operate within a closed system, we are doomed to regress. If we enlarge our awareness to include social, economic, and political factors; admit new information from a variety of sources; take advantage of the capacity to integrate past and present perceptions and concepts, we will leap forward.

—E. M. GILFOYLE (1984, P. 576)

W hy write about unique clinical practice and innovative ideas in occupational therapy? The *Centennial Vision* of the American Occupational Therapy Association (AOTA, 2007) envisioned the profession at its 100-year mark as being "widely recognized, science-driven, and evidence-based" (p. 613), and practitioners who describe novel interventions for a wider audience contribute to the realization of this vision. The profession is more *widely recognized* when the public has access to persuasive information by practitioners about their unique clinical practice and innovative ideas.

In addition, describing innovative practice in scholarly publications promotes a *science-driven* and *evidence-based* profession; this activity has been referred to as the *scholarship of practice* (AOTA, 2009). Thus, writing about unique clinical practice and innovative ideas allows others to understand the richness and diversity of occupational therapy, enables other practitioners to apply these ideas, supports a wider array of clients served, and fosters growth of the profession.

This chapter introduces the process of writing about a creative and innovative occupational therapy program or service. Many creative and innovative programs and services have been developed, but to bring benefits to the profession as a whole, practitioners involved must describe their efforts skillfully and persuasively and publicly disseminate the written product.

This chapter provides exercises (see Box 12.1) to develop practitioners' thinking about a unique practice in preparation for writing about it and a three-step process to structure that writing. Each step of the process is illustrated using the case of Michele, an occupational therapist with more than 25 years of clinical experience in adult rehabilitation services and an innovative idea for helping her clients who have experienced traumatic brain injury (TBI).

Case Presentation: Michele

Michele developed a clinical training model using portable personal electronic devices to support clients who have substantial memory loss following a TBI. This innovative approach was very successful, but it required the client to have the financial resources to purchase the electronic device. For many clients, this was an extreme financial burden. Michele had been effective in appealing to philanthropic groups to purchase devices for clients who faced financial hardships, but she felt that third-party payers should be purchasing the devices. Her dilemma was how to convince these third-party payers to do so. She had written numerous letters to third-party payers requesting payment and documenting client improvements from using these electronic devices as a support for memory, but these requests were denied.

As Michele considered her dilemma, she posed two questions. First, how could she convince third-party payers to purchase these devices? Second, how could she inform other occupational therapy practitioners about the advantages of using these devices with their clients?

BOX 12.1.
FIVE EXERCISES TO FOSTER WRITING ABOUT A UNIQUE CLINICAL PRACTICE OR INNOVATIVE SERVICE

1. Identify an occupational therapy topic area that interests you or in which you have experience.
   - Is this topic well established within the profession? How many years?
   - Is it an emerging topic? Are others engaged in this topic?
   - What specific issues within the topic intrigue you? Subdivide the larger topic into smaller segments.
2. Identify what you know about the topic and how you know that information.
   - Is your knowledge base broad or limited in scope?
   - How much of your knowledge is based on personal experiences?
   - How much of your knowledge is based on published information?
3. Compare your knowledge base with published information.
   - Search the literature, and compare your knowledge base with the published information.
   - What are the specific similarities and differences?
   - Even if there are only slight differences, your knowledge base can add to the body of knowledge about the topic: This is what you should write about!
4. Identify how your knowledge base can contribute to the profession.
   - Does this information expand basic understanding of a topic (e.g., unique occupational characteristics of a client group)?
   - Does this information describe intervention methods (e.g., specific outcomes of innovative services)?
   - Could this information contribute to policy changes that could advance the profession?
5. Identify the most likely audience who would benefit from reading an article about this topic.
   - Would this information be best used by occupational therapy practitioners in a specific practice area, such as Special Interest Section members, or would a wider audience benefit from this information through an article in *OT Practice* or *Today in OT*?
   - What background information does this audience need to fully appreciate the information you can provide?
   - What are the two or three key points you need to make about this specific topic? These should be addressed in both your introduction and your conclusion.

Writing About Unique Clinical Practice and Innovative Ideas

The process of writing about unique clinical practice and innovative ideas can be divided into three steps:

1. Orient the audience to the context and environment. Who will most likely read this information? What do readers need to know about the larger social, cultural, and physical environment in which the service or program is positioned? What literature currently exists about the setting and available services?
2. Provide a clear demonstration of need.
3. Describe the new service or program developed to address the need and explain how it meets that need. What are the differences between the context and intervention information in the available literature and those of the innovative service or program? What is the message readers should take away?

This approach of identifying the circumstances, describing the need, and explaining the new way to meet the need has frequently been used in the evidence-based literature. Two articles illustrate this approach: one describing a new way to promote social skills in children with autism and the other describing a yoga intervention for third graders.

Wong and Kwan's (2010) discussion of a program to foster social interaction in children who have autism can be summarized as follows:

1. The authors began by describing the problems children who have autism face in settings that require social interaction and the limitations of currently available services. They reviewed the literature on typical services designed to foster social interaction in children with autism, which often require intensive intervention of many hours a week over a lengthy period of time, often several years. They noted that the effectiveness of the current model had recently been called into question.
2. They highlighted the need for a less costly model with demonstrated effectiveness.
3. They explained how their program differed from current models; instead of lengthy intervention services, the new program was of a short duration (2 weeks) and trained parents and caregivers to foster social skills development during short but frequent daily sessions. The authors offered evidence of the benefits of this approach for the children, including gains in social skills.

Case-Smith, Sines, and Klatt (2010) provided another example of the three-step process in an article on yoga instruction for third-grade students from low socioeconomic status (SES) backgrounds to reduce stress and improve classroom behavior. They first provided a social context by describing the stress faced by school-age children from low-SES backgrounds. Second, they described the need by noting the negative effects of this stress on the children's behavior and their ability to participate in the learning environment. Third, they noted that the use of yoga as a stress reduction method had been documented in other settings and that they used this approach in a novel situation, a public school, and with an underserved group—children of low SES. They showed how their 8-week yoga program provided by occupational therapy students within the school helped children feel more calm and focused, promoted better control of their personal behavior, and improved their self-concept.

ORIENT THE AUDIENCE TO THE CONTEXT AND ENVIRONMENT

When occupational therapy practitioners document client services in clinical practice, the focus of their writing is on the client's occupational needs, the intervention services provided, and the outcome of those services (Sames, 2010). Typically, information about the context and environment is embedded in clinical documentation but not fully described. For example, if a practitioner is discussing changes in client performance of self-care skills within an acute care setting, he or she provides only limited description of the social and physical environment. Likewise, a practitioner documenting client progress in an outpatient hand clinic does not provide lengthy descriptions of the environment. The writer of a clinical documentation note assumes that readers, typically physicians or third-party payers, understand the context and environment.

Occupational therapy practitioners working in novel settings or with innovative practices who wish to describe their work effectively need to expand their foundational clinical documentation skills to describe the unique elements of the situation, particularly the context and environment. For example, when working with families who are homeless and living in a shelter, it would be important to describe the physical setting and the cultural expectations before discussing unique occupational therapy services provided to this population (Schultz-Krohn, Drnek, & Powell, 2006). The practitioner needs to position the innovative practice within a contextual framework to allow readers to understand not only the intervention being provided but also the clinical reasoning behind it. This detail sets the stage for the description of the innovative practice.

As the writer sets the stage, he or she needs to answer the following questions:

1. What is the larger social, cultural, and physical environment where the specific setting or innovative service is positioned?
2. What is currently known about the setting and typically provided services? This answer may be very brief if no literature is found.
3. How do the context and environment of the innovative service or program differ from currently available information?

The *Occupational Therapy Practice Framework: Domain and Process* (AOTA, 2008) can guide you in writing about the details of the context and environment. Before beginning to write, search the literature and determine what is known about the physical, social, cultural, and personal elements of the area of interest. If that information is available in the literature, explain how your setting or services are either similar to or different than what has been described. For example, most shelters for homeless families are designed exclusively for mothers with young children, typically ages 6 years or younger (Rog & Buckner, 2007). Providing services in a shelter where families include fathers, husbands, boyfriends, and teenagers represents a situation that differs from what is typically described in the literature addressing shelter services for homeless families (Schultz-Krohn, 2004). The practitioner must clearly describe this contextual information, which represents the unique social environment of this setting, for readers before explaining the details of the occupational therapy services provided.

Before beginning to write, search the literature and determine what is known about the physical, social, cultural, and personal elements of the area of interest. If that information is available in the literature, explain how your setting or services are either similar to or different than what has been described.

Let's return to Michele. As she began to write about her innovative method to help clients who had sustained a TBI, she turned to the *Framework* to help organize her writing. In a draft letter to third-party payers, Michele described the current practices used with clients who have sustained a TBI and have significant memory loss. She explained that these clients typically require supervision when they engage in community activities such as grocery shopping or going to the movies. The social environment thus includes another person serving as a memory aid for the client, and if that support person is not available, the client faces challenges to participation. She also described how the general public (social environment) regularly uses technology memory supports. Many individuals routinely use cell phone calendars or other electronic organizers as a reminder of appointments.

This background set the stage for Michele's explanation of how her innovative program could meet these needs. Michele had already seen the benefits of using the electronic devices to support her clients, but in previous attempts to obtain the devices for her clients she had not positioned that information within the context and environment of the larger community.

DEMONSTRATE THE NEED

The second step in describing an innovation is to clearly identify the clinical need or problem. When writing about a unique clinical practice or innovative service, you need to identify current knowledge about a problem or need. The current literature may provide background information and identify similar problems or issues, strengthening the description of the unique clinical practice or innovative approach. A needs assessment is a systematic approach to gathering information about a specific group or population that can be provided to those who can make changes in policy and programs to serve the specific group or population (Finlayson, 2006). The needs assessment process can serve as a structure to organize writing about a unique clinical practice or innovative service.

The four steps outlined for a needs assessment are

1. Identify the specific issues related to the real world.
2. Consider who would best use this information.
3. Examine the political orientation of the unique clinical practice or innovative service.
4. Understand the scope of the problem (local vs. broad national or global concerns).

In any writing about unique clinical practice or innovative services, the author must consider and address these four elements. The needs assessment approach typically includes asking those directly involved with the situation to provide information, similar to developing an occupational profile with a client (AOTA, 2008). The client is best able to describe the problems and issues that compromise his or her occupational performance.

EXPLAIN HOW THE INNOVATION MEETS THE NEED

The third step, explaining how the innovation meets the need, is the most critical. Some writers begin the writing process with this step; you may first identify the two or three important messages you wish to convey to your audience and focus your discussion of the first two points to address the importance of your message. In this way, your description of the context and environmental features of the novel clinical practice or service will provide enough details to directly address the actual purpose of the writing. The focus is to deliver useable information about the novel clinical practice or innovative service.

As she described the context and environment of her innovative idea, Michele kept the perspective of her audience, specifically the insurance reviewer, in mind. From an insurance perspective, services need to be both effective and cost-effective. Michele needed not only to justify the effectiveness of the intervention she had proposed but also to explain how this new intervention would both benefit the client and meet the need of the insurance reviewer to contain costs. Michele had provided loaner electronic devices to four clients who were unable to secure funding through their insurance companies. She asked these clients to write a letter indicating how the electronic device allowed them greater access to the community with reduced dependence on the personal attendant or family member. This greater freedom reduced the amount of time the insurance company needed to pay for an attendant. Although the insurance company still needed to pay for supportive personal attendants, the number of hours could be slightly reduced, resulting in a cost savings.

The Next Step: Publishing

Michele was able to successfully convince one insurer to purchase an electronic memory aid for her client. This success prompted Michele to consider how she could promote system-wide change to support other clients who sustained a TBI. She realized that she needed to share her success in obtaining funding for her client to receive electronic memory devices with other occupational therapy practitioners. Although she had not completed a traditionally designed research project, she felt that practitioners would benefit from knowing about her use of electronic memory devices and her ability to obtain funding for these devices.

She looked at options for publicly disseminating this information. She presented a poster session at her state occupational therapy association conference, but only those in attendance had an opportunity to view this information. She looked at AOTA's Special Interest Section newsletters and *OT Practice,* both of which regularly publish short articles about innovative practice. Michele realized that practitioners working in the area of geriatrics, mental health, and physical disabilities might be interested in the use of these devices and in the process she used to obtain funding. She contacted the editor of *OT Practice* to obtain the submission requirements.

Michele then began the process of writing about her unique approach to memory problems for clients who have sustained a TBI. She started by identifying two key points she wanted to convey in the article: first, that the use of electronic memory devices was both beneficial to clients and cost-effective, and second, that effectively presenting these benefits in writing could convince third-party payers to fund the devices. These points served as her focus for the article. She used the three guiding questions to support the process of writing: What do readers need to know about the situation, context, and environment? What is the clinical problem or need? And how does this innovation meet the need? In her draft, Michele described the frequency and consequences of memory loss for clients who sustained a TBI. She explained that third-party payers typically were reluctant to purchase electronic memory aids for clients. She discussed not only the evidence that this device helped clients who had sustained a TBI but also the process she used to obtain funding.

After several revisions, the article was near completion. Michele asked an occupational therapy professor with whom she had remained in contact for feedback on her work. The professor offered specific suggestions to strengthen the article and polished

> **The three guiding questions to support the process of writing: What do readers need to know about the situation, context, and environment? What is the clinical problem or need? And how does this innovation meet the need?**

her reference citations. Michele used the feedback to complete the article and submitted it to *OT Practice*, which published it!

Michele reflected on the process of not only securing funding for her client but also taking the time to publish an article. At first she had considered the process of writing to be outside the practice of occupational therapy unless directly related to documenting client services. She now realized that when occupational therapy practitioners publicly demonstrate the effectiveness of occupational therapy services, the profession is recognized and grows. Publishing her article in *OT Practice* brought an additional benefit: She was able to use the publication when writing letters of justification to third-party payers to secure funding for other clients.

Spreading the Word About Unique Clinical Practice and Innovative Services

Writing about unique clinical practice and innovative services is an important part of occupational therapy practitioners' professional responsibilities. To support the AOTA *Centennial Vision* of the profession as "widely recognized, science-driven, and evidence-based," practitioners need to make their innovations publicly accessible to fellow professionals, third-party payers, and all those who might benefit from occupational therapy services.

REFERENCES

American Occupational Therapy Association. (2007). AOTA's *Centennial Vision* and executive summary. *American Journal of Occupational Therapy, 61,* 613–614. doi:10.5014/ajot.61.6.613

American Occupational Therapy Association. (2008). Occupational therapy practice framework: Domain and process (2nd ed.). *American Journal of Occupational Therapy, 62,* 625–683. doi:10.5014/ajot.62.6.625

American Occupational Therapy Association. (2009). Scholarship in occupational therapy. *American Journal of Occupational Therapy, 63,* 790–796. doi:10.5014/ajot.63.6.790

Case-Smith, J., Sines, J. S., & Klatt, M. (2010). Perceptions of children who participated in a school-based yoga program. *Journal of Occupational Therapy, Schools, and Early Intervention, 3,* 226–238.

Finlayson, M. (2006). Assessing need for services. In G. Keilhofner (Ed.), *Research in occupational therapy* (pp. 591–606). Philadelphia: F. A. Davis.

Gilfoyle, E. M. (1984). Transformation of a profession (Eleanor Clarke Slagle Lecture). *American Journal of Occupational Therapy, 38,* 575–584.

Rog, D. J., & Buckner, J. C. (2007, March). Homeless families and children. In D. Dennis, G. Locke, & J. Khadduri (Eds.), *Toward understanding homelessness: The 2007 National Symposium on Homelessness Research.* Washington, DC: U.S. Department of Health and Human Services, U.S. Department of Housing and Urban Development. Retrieved August 3, 2011, from http://aspe.hhs.gov/hsp/homelessness/symposium07/rog

Sames, K. (2010). *Documenting occupational therapy practice* (2nd ed.). Upper Saddle River, NJ: Prentice Hall.

Schultz-Krohn, W. A. (2004). The meaning of family routines in a homeless shelter. *American Journal of Occupational Therapy, 58,* 531–542. doi:10.5014/ajot.58.5.531

Schultz-Krohn, W., Drnek, S., & Powell, K. (2006). Occupational therapy intervention to foster goal-setting skills for homeless mothers. *Occupational Therapy in Health Care, 20,* 149–166.

Wong, V. C., & Kwan, Q. K. (2010). Randomized controlled trial for early intervention for autism: A pilot study of Autism 1-2-3 project. *Journal of Autism and Developmental Disorders, 40,* 667–688.

ADDITIONAL RESOURCES

Chan, J. F., & Lutovich, D. (2003). *Professional writing skills: A self-paced training program.* San Anselmo, CA: Advanced Communication Designs.

Galvan, J. L. (2006). *Writing literature reviews* (3rd ed.). Glendale, CA: Pyrczak.

Gurdon, M. (2008). *Write on! The no-nonsense guide to professional writing.* London: New Holland.

Hacker, D. (2008). *A writer's reference* (6th ed.). Boston: Bedford/St. Martin's.

13

Documenting Occupational Therapy Services

JERILYN (GIGI) SMITH, MS, OTR/L, SWC

My task, which I am trying to achieve is, by the power of the written word, to make you hear, to make you feel—it is, before all, to make you see.

—Joseph Conrad, *Lord Jim*

Documentation is seldom regarded as a favorite aspect of the therapy process. Accurate, efficient, and professionally written documentation, however, is a key component of occupational therapy practice. The American Occupational Therapy Association (AOTA, 2008a) identified the purposes of documentation as being to

- Articulate the rationale for provision of occupational therapy services and the relationship of services to the client's outcome
- Reflect the practitioner's clinical reasoning and professional judgment
- Communicate information about the client from the occupational therapy perspective
- Create a chronological record of client status, occupational therapy services provided to the client, and client outcomes.

Documentation is required whenever occupational therapy services are delivered. It provides a forum for practitioners to explain what happened in the therapy session and to demonstrate the clinical reasoning they used to guide the therapy process. Documentation is the means by which practitioners inform payer sources about what occurs in occupational therapy, and well-written documentation is crucial for reimbursement of services. This chapter describes elements of effective documentation, types of occupational therapy documentation, reimbursement requirements, legal and ethical concerns, and issues in electronic documentation.

Elements of Effective Documentation

Effective documentation is concise yet complete and includes all of the relevant information necessary without being wordy or redundant. As in all professional written communication, proper grammar and correct spelling are essential, and all handwritten entries must be legible. Jargon (i.e., language or acronyms unique to occupational therapy) may be meaningless or misunderstood by non–occupational therapy practitioners and should be avoided in documentation.

Use of the active voice is preferred over the passive voice (Online Writing Laboratory at Purdue University, 2010; Sames, 2010). A sentence using the active voice states the subject of the sentence, making clear who performed the action. In a sentence using passive voice, the subject of the sentence is not specified, leaving readers wondering who performed the action. "Clients in the social skills group were provided with an orientation session" is an example of the passive voice, whereas "The group leader provided an orientation session to clients attending the social skills group" is an example of the active voice.

The following fundamentals of documentation are important to adhere to when writing in the medical record (AOTA, 2008a):

- The client's full name appears on each page of documentation.
- The date of service is specified.
- The type of documentation, agency, and department are identified.
- Only the practitioner providing the intervention writes notes. It is considered fraudulent to write a note for another practitioner or to change the wording in another professional's written documentation.

- All entries are signed by the practitioner performing the intervention. Signatures include, at minimum, the practitioner's first name or initial, last name, and professional designation (e.g., OTR/L, OT/L, OTA, COTA). The practitioner must be aware of and abide by state regulations regarding the use of professional designations.
- An occupational therapist countersigns documentation by students and occupational therapy assistants in accordance with reimbursement or state regulations.
- Terminology used is acceptable as defined by the setting. Only approved abbreviations are used (see Boxes 13.1 and 13.2).
- The record describes the action, behavior, or signs and symptoms the practitioner observed. Information obtained from others (e.g., nurse, family member, caregiver) is clearly indicated, and quotations are used when appropriate. Judgmental statements and assumptions are not included.
- Practitioners correct errors by drawing a single line through the word or sentence, initialing and dating in the margin, and writing "error." Correction fluid is never used, and entries are never erased or obliterated, as this may appear to be an attempt to prevent others from knowing what was originally written.
- Late entries to the medical record are identified in the margin as "late entry" and dated.
- Words or sentences have not been squeezed into existing text; doing so might be interpreted as adding missing information or supplementing existing information to support something that happened after the original documentation was completed. Although no fraudulent intent may be present, the content could be interpreted as such if it were ever called into question (Smith, 2013).
- No blank spaces are left on preprinted forms or at the end of a narrative note. If the writing does not extend to the end of the line, a single line is drawn that extends from the last word in the sentence to the end of the line. If it is not appropriate to address a particular area on a form, "n/a" is inserted to indicate that these areas were not appropriate to assess and were not overlooked.
- Confidentiality standards are upheld.
- Professional standards of technology are adhered to.
- Records are disposed of according to law or agency requirements.
- Agency or legal requirements for storage of records are complied with.

BOX 13.1.

COMMON ABBREVIATIONS FOR CLINICAL DOCUMENTATION

A	assessment	h, hr	hour
Add	adduction	min	minute
ADL	activities of daily living	MP, MCP	metacarpophalangeal joint
adm	admission, admitted	NPO	nothing by mouth
AE	above elbow	PH	past history
AFO	ankle–foot–orthosis	PIP	proximal interphalangeal
AK	above knee		joint
a.m.	morning	p.m.	afternoon
ant	anterior	PMH	past medical history
AP	anterior–posterior	p.o.	by mouth, orally
AROM	active range of motion	post.	posterior
assist	assistance, assistive	PROM	passive range of motion
BE	below elbow	Pt., pt.	patient
BM	bowel movement	PTA	prior to admission
BOS	base of support	PWB	partial weight bearing
BR	bedrest	q	every
B/S	bedside	qd	every day
cal	calories	qh	every hour
c/o	complains of	qid	four times a day
cont.	continue	qn	every night
D/C	discontinued or discharged	R	right
dept.	department	re:	regarding
DIP	distal interphalangeal joint	rehab	rehabilitation
DNR	do not resuscitate	reps	repetitions
DOB	date of birth	R/O	rule out
DOE	dyspnea on exertion	ROM	range of motion
Dx	diagnosis	RR	respiratory rate
ECF	extended care facility	RROM	resistive range of motion
eob	edge of bed	RUE	right upper extremity
eval.	evaluation	Rx	intervention plan, therapy
ex	exercise	sec	seconds
ext.	extension	SLR	straight leg raise
FH	family history	SNF	skilled nursing facility
flex.	flexion	SOB	short of breath
FWB	full weight bearing	S/P	status post
fx	fracture	stat	immediately

BOX 13.1.
COMMON ABBREVIATIONS FOR CLINICAL DOCUMENTATION *(cont.)*

sup	superior	UE	upper extremity
Sx	symptoms	VC	vital capacity
ther ex	therapeutic exercise	v.o.	verbal orders
tid	three times daily	v.s.	vital signs
TKR	total knee replacement	WBAT	weight bearing as
t.o.	telephone order		tolerated
TTWB	toe touch weight bearing	w/c	wheelchair
Tx	treatment	WNL	within normal limits

Source. Kettenbach (2004).

BOX 13.2.
COMMON ABBREVIATIONS FOR EDUCATION-RELATED DOCUMENTATION

APE	adapted physical education
AT	assistive technology
CFR	*Code of Federal Regulations*
DOE	Department of Education
ECFE	early childhood family education
ECSE	early childhood special education
EI	early intervention
IDEA	Individuals With Disabilities Education Act
IEP	individualized education program
IFSP	individualized family service plan
LD	learning disability
LRE	least restrictive environment
OHI	other health impaired
PI	physically impaired
PLEP	present level of educational performance
SEA	state education agency
SI	sensory integration

Sources. Jackson (2007); Sames (2010).

Documentation should use the terminology outlined in the *Occupational Therapy Practice Framework: Domain and Process* (AOTA, 2008b). The *Framework* provides language that is appropriate to use in describing the results of the client evaluation, interventions, and outcomes and that communicates occupational therapy's unique focus on occupation and daily life activities to other professionals, consumers of services, and third-party payers. Documentation should include factors that influence performance (performance skills, performance patterns, activity demands, client factors, and context and environment). The practitioner observes and analyzes performance skills in order to understand the underlying factors that support or hinder engagement in occupational performance, and this analysis is included in the written record.

Professional reasoning (also called *clinical reasoning* or *therapeutic reasoning*) is the process clinicians use to plan, direct, perform, and reflect on client care (Schell, 2009). Documentation must demonstrate that the clinician used professional reasoning in the decision-making process during all aspects of the client's therapy program. *Scientific reasoning* is used in understanding the client's condition, impairments, and disabilities; in determining how these might influence occupational performance; and in deciding on interventions that are in the client's best interest. Clinicians use *narrative reasoning* to understand the client's life story and evaluate the meaning occupational performance deficits might have for the client. *Pragmatic reasoning* is used when addressing the practical realities associated with the delivery of therapy services—for example, when the practitioner evaluates resources for intervention, considers reimbursement restraints and practice trends, and incorporates this information into documentation. *Ethical reasoning* is used in deciding on the most appropriate therapy intervention to address the client's occupational performance needs (Schell, 2009). Professional reasoning skills enhance not only client care but also the effectiveness of documentation and ultimately reimbursement for therapy services.

> **Professional reasoning skills enhance not only client care but also the effectiveness of documentation and ultimately reimbursement for therapy services.**

Types of Occupational Therapy Documentation

Time spent in documentation typically is not reimbursable, so efficiency is essential. The use of checklists and forms that reduce the need for narrative writing can reduce lost productivity from time spent in documentation. Practitioners in many settings use flow sheets and checklists in conjunction with SOAP notes and narrative notes (discussed later in this section). For example, a flow sheet may be used to record daily status, and a longer, more comprehensive note may be written weekly to summarize progress. Succinct, clear, and accurate documentation that keeps the target audience in mind will ensure that relevant information is conveyed to the health care team and facilitate reimbursement for therapy services.

Documentation is an ongoing process that often begins even before the client evaluation takes place and continues throughout the therapy program. Places where occupational therapy practitioners document include screening reports, initial and reevaluation reports, progress notes, transition plan reports, discharge summaries, other medical record entries (e.g., interdisciplinary notes, care plans, physician telephone orders, treatment clarification orders), treatment and equipment authorization requests, professional communications between members of the health care team, home programs and reports to families and other health care professionals, and outcome data reports. This section discusses two categories of reports in detail: evaluation reports and intervention reports.

EVALUATION REPORTS

The initial evaluation is the foundation for the client's therapy program and contains both objective and subjective information. According to the *Framework,* the evaluation focuses on "finding out what the client wants and needs to do, determining what the client can do and has done, and identifying those factors that act as supports or barriers to health and participation" (AOTA, 2008b, p. 649). A detailed accounting of the client's current status as well as a description of his or her prior status is necessary to justify the need for occupational therapy services and to establish a baseline from which to formulate goals and measure progress.

The evaluation consists of the occupational therapy profile and an analysis of occupational performance. Information obtained during the interview for the occupational profile guides the practitioner in deciding on appropriate assessments, interventions, and goals. The analysis of occupational performance entails collecting and interpreting information using standardized and nonstandardized assessments and skilled clinical observation of the client's performance in activities related to desired occupations. Clinical judgment skills are used to determine which assessments are the most appropriate to evaluate the client's occupational needs, problems, and concerns. Clinical judgment is also used in documenting the analysis of the client's occupational performance and assessment results to identify what supports and what hinders client performance. The practitioner then develops goals and an intervention plan in collaboration with the client and records them in the written evaluation report. Justification for services is dependent on the initial evaluation reports, so it is critical that documentation clearly and comprehensively cover all areas necessary to support the need for therapy services.

INTERVENTION REPORTS

One of the expectations of occupational therapy intervention is that the client will make progress in attaining goals. Progress toward goals is necessary for reimbursement purposes and to justify continued services. Well-written intervention reports (often called *progress notes*) clearly demonstrate the client's progress or, if there is none, identify the reasons why progress was not made. Depending on reimbursement and practice setting requirements, progress reports may be written daily, weekly, and/or monthly. Shorter contact notes may be required in some settings; contact notes record the services provided during the session and the client's response rather than progress (Brennan & Robinson, 2006). All notes should be written as close to the time of the client contact as possible to improve accuracy and to ensure that notes are in chronological order in the client record.

Several different formats may be used to document client response to intervention, including SOAP notes and narrative notes (discussed in the two subsections that follow) and checklists. Regardless of the format used, progress reports should include the following key elements related to the intervention session:

- Results of the intervention (outcomes) using terminology from the *Framework* and including objective measurements

- Skilled interventions the practitioner provided
- A statement of measurable progress toward identified goals
- The practitioner's clinical judgments and subjective impressions
- The plan for future sessions.

The practitioner's professional (clinical) reasoning that influenced the choice of the intervention used should also be reflected in the progress report. The practitioner modifies and updates goals on the basis of the client's progress.

SOAP Notes

The SOAP note was first introduced by Dr. Lawrence Weed in 1970 as a part of the problem-oriented medical record (POMR) model (Weed, 1971). In the POMR, the clinician creates a numbered list of the client's unique problems. All members of the health care team write a SOAP note to address the problems in the list that are specific to their area of expertise. SOAP is an acronym, with each letter standing for the name of a section in the note: S = *subjective,* O = *objective,* A = *assessment,* and P = *plan.*

In the subjective (S) section of the note, the practitioner includes information reported by the client, family, caregiver, or others involved with the client and gives the perspective of each on the client's condition or treatment. Subjective data cannot be measured or verified during the treatment session. The client's subjective response to treatment is also recorded in this section of the note. Information such as expressions of feelings, attitudes, concerns, fatigue, pain, goals, or plans (Borcherding, 2005) is appropriate to include in the S section. Direct quotes are often used. If the client is nonverbal, gestures, facial expressions, and other types of nonverbal responses can be included.

Practitioners should include only subjective statements that are relevant to the therapeutic intervention in the subjective section. They should avoid including statements that can be misinterpreted, that might jeopardize reimbursement, or that do not relate to the intervention session. Subjective statements should also relate to information in other parts of the note. The client's statements can be summarized if necessary to increase the clarity of the note.

Examples of S statements include the following:

- Client reports he has always coughed when drinking water.
- "I get anxious whenever I have to make a decision."
- "I can't remember what step comes next."
- Parent reports that J screams whenever his hair is washed.

- Client reports pain in his right arm following therapy session yesterday.
- Mother reports that L's teacher states L cannot sit in chair without fidgeting.

In the objective (O) section of the SOAP note, the practitioner reports the measurable results of assessments and objective observations (Ketterbach, 2004). Examples of measurable information include muscle grades, range-of-motion measurements, performance levels of assistance (Table 13.1), pain scale measurements, number of repetitions, amount of time, number of times, distance, quality of movement, and task completion.

TABLE 13.1. Performance Levels of Assistance

Performance Level	Description
Independence	Client is completely independent.
	Client requires no physical or verbal assistance to complete the task.
	Client completes task safely.
Modified independence	Client is completely independent with task but may require additional time or adaptive equipment.
Supervision	Client requires supervision to safely complete task.
	Client may require a verbal cue for safety.
Contact guard, standby assistance	Hands-on, contact guard assistance is necessary for client to safely complete the task, or caregiver must be within arm's length for safety.
Minimum assistance	Client requires up to 25% physical or verbal assistance[a] by one person to safely complete the task.
Moderate assistance	Client requires 26% to 50% physical or verbal assistance[a] by one person to safely complete the task.
Maximal assistance	Client requires 51% to 75% physical or verbal assistance[a] by one person to safely complete the task.
Dependence	Client requires more than 75% assistance to complete the task.

[a]It is important to state whether assistance provided is physical or verbal.

Only factual information and observed behaviors are included in this section. The *Framework* provides a structure for identifying the areas that can be addressed. Aspects of the occupational therapy domain include client factors, performance skills, performance patterns, context and environment, and activity demands. Results of standardized and nonstandardized assessments, measurable performance of functional tasks (e.g., basic and instrumental activities of daily living [ADLs], play, leisure, education, work and social participation), coordination, movement patterns, activity tolerance, posture and balance, functional mobility, and endurance are examples of areas that might be reported on in the objective section. Other appropriate areas to discuss in this section include cognitive functions, psychosocial factors (e.g., mood, affect, ability to engage with others), social interaction (e.g., awareness of others, initiation of conversation, interaction with peers), appearance (e.g., grooming, hygiene, attire), behavior (e.g., agitation, affect, impulsivity, safety awareness, anxiety), judgment and problem solving, and ability to follow directions (Borcherding, 2005). A description of the intervention should precede the summary of what the practitioner observed. The practitioner does not analyze or interpret the data in the objective section of the SOAP note; only objective descriptions of the client's performance are included.

Examples of O statements include the following:

- PROM testing RUE—full PROM at shoulder, elbow, and wrist; 0°–50° MP flexion, 0°–30° PIP and DIP flexion [see Box 13.1 for abbreviations].
- During upper-body dressing training, client required moderate assistance to don T-shirt because of difficulty orienting shirt to body and sequencing the task. Client required moderate verbal assistance for problem solving and minimal assistance for sitting balance at edge of bed during activity.
- Socialization group: Client initiated conversation with 2 other group members without verbal cuing from group leader. She had moderate difficulty staying on task during the structured activity and required frequent redirection to complete task (making a collage).
- Feeding training: Client was able to feed self 100% of meal with minimal assistance (verbal) to use strategies (chin tuck, head turn, double swallow) for safe eating.
- Fine motor coordination training: Client was able to use tripod grasp to pick up small, round objects on 2/5 attempts. Client preferred using raking motion to retrieve objects.

In the assessment (A) section of the SOAP note, the practitioner uses clinical reasoning to interpret the information from the S and O sections. He or she analyzes the client's strengths, impairments, and functional deficits to determine what impact they have on occupational performance. The practitioner summarizes relevant assessment findings and results of performance, synthesizes these findings, analyzes the impact any deficits have on the client's ability to engage in meaningful occupations, and formulates the intervention plan for future therapy sessions. In this section the practitioner demonstrates how clinical reasoning is used to guide the intervention process.

Borcherding (2005) suggested organizing the analysis of the S and O information in the A section of the note by addressing three areas: problems, progress, and rehabilitation potential. *Problems* may include safety concerns, problem-solving and coping strategy deficits, areas of function that are not within normal limits, and inconsistencies between the client report and the objective findings. *Progress* toward identified goals demonstrates that treatment is effective and can be reported using a comparison statement—for example, "Client now dons shoes independently (last week he required minimal assistance)." A lack of progress should also be explained in the A section. *Rehabilitation potential* is described on the basis of an analysis of what is reported in the S and O sections and clinical judgment and reflects the client's ability to meet the stated objectives and benefit from ongoing therapy services.

Examples of A statements include the following:

- T exhibits difficulties with abstract thinking but understands concrete ideas. She also shows deficits in short-term memory, but she now recognizes that she requires assistance for her memory problems; last week she was unaware of this. T will benefit from continued skilled intervention to develop strategies for her memory loss to allow her to be safe alone at home for short periods of time.
- Although B came to group without complaint (last week he refused to come), he appeared to want to draw attention with negative comments and argumentative behavior. B followed instructions but exhibited a defiant attitude by drawing only in black ink and refusing offers of colored markers or photos for his collage. Progress was noted in B's attendance in group and his cooperativeness in following directions. He will benefit from further occupational therapy to continue working on positive social interaction with peers.

- G shows good improvement in shoulder active ROM (he now has 0°–70° active shoulder flexion; last week he had 0°–60°). Pain and stiffness in the morning continue to be limiting factors for ADL independence. Because of limitations in AROM and pain, G cannot independently don his shirt. He is making good gains, however, and with continued therapy, AROM should continue to increase. G will benefit from additional techniques to decrease stiffness and pain.

The last section of the SOAP note is the plan (P). The practitioner continually revises the plan as the client meets the stated short-term goals and updated short-term goals are established. As appropriate to the client's progress or the development of new problems, additional interventions or referrals to other services are introduced in this section.

Examples of P statements include the following:

- Continue daily occupational therapy services for ADL training and instruction in compensatory strategies to increase client's independence in dressing to supervised level.
- Continue with weekly occupational therapy. Emphasize taking turns, making socially appropriate responses, and respecting personal boundaries in a social peer group setting. Short-term goal: Client will respect personal boundaries by not touching other group members and will not display any socially inappropriate responses during the group activity. She will wait her turn during group discussion with minimal cues from the group leader.

Figure 13.1 is an example of a progress note using the SOAP format.

Although SOAP notes are not used in every practice setting, the SOAP format is an excellent one to assist practitioners in evaluating the client's performance from several perspectives. The available data can then be analyzed to determine the best plan of action to achieve meaningful client goals. Although the content will vary depending on the type of therapy setting, third-party payer requirements, and client needs, the *subjective, objective, assessment,* and *plan* categories provide a useful structure for well-written documentation.

> Although the content will vary depending on the type of therapy setting, third-party payer requirements, and client needs, the *subjective, objective, assessment,* and *plan* categories provide a useful structure for well-written documentation.

Subjective

Client reports, "It takes too much energy to dress each day, and I'm not able to use any of the equipment you gave me." Client also states that upper extremity (UE) stiffness makes it difficult to dress. Client's husband reports that client seems discouraged because she needs help with dressing tasks and will not get dressed unless she has a doctor's appointment.

Objective

Client requires moderate assistance to use dressing stick and shoehorn for lower body dressing (last week she was dependent). She requires minimal assistance with fitted blouse (last week she required moderate assistance). She is unable to button blouse even with buttonhook. Client became short of breath during seated self-care task (dressing) after 5 min of activity.

Assessment

Client is improving in her ability to complete the self-care task of dressing; however, she is having difficulty remembering how to use the adaptive equipment, which impedes her independence. Stiffness in her shoulders interferes with reaching and independence. Joint changes in both hands make functional grasp difficult. Chronic obstructive pulmonary disease still interferes with client's ability to independently and efficiently complete activity of daily living (ADL) tasks.

Plan

- Continue ADL training with emphasis on adaptive equipment use. Provide written directions for equipment use. Assess ability to don looser, over-the-head blouse.
- Instruct client in fatigue management techniques, including pursed lip breathing, during dressing.
- Instruct client in active range of motion exercises to use before beginning morning ADL routine to decrease UE stiffness.

FIGURE 13.1. Sample SOAP note.

Narrative Notes

In many settings the narrative note is used to document the results of the intervention session. Narrative notes may be written either directly into the client's medical record or in a designated therapy section of the client's chart. If the note is written directly into the client record, it must be entered in chronological order, and in many settings, the time that the note was written in addition to the time of the intervention session must be recorded (Fremgen, 2009). A narrative note conveys information that supports the need for the intervention. One way to organize a narrative note is to categorize the information into three subsections:

1. *Description of program:* "FBL was seen for 30 min for lower body dressing training."
2. *Results of intervention and client's response, highlighting progress:* "FBL required moderate assistance to lean forward to reach his feet while seated at the edge of the bed (last week FBL required maximal assistance). Weight bearing was facilitated at the pelvis to improve stabilization for balance shifts. FBL required maximal assistance to position pant leg over foot secondary to sequencing and perceptual deficits (FBL was dependent for this component of the task last week). Sit to stand with moderate assistance (maximal assist last week), and maximal assistance required (dependent last week) to hike pants. FBL required frequent rest periods secondary to shortness of breath with activity. FBL has made good progress this week."
3. *Plan for future intervention sessions:* "Continue daily dressing training with emphasis on facilitation of balance responses during lower body dressing, establish a consistent routine and sequence of task components, and use tactile cues for left neglect. Initiate training for donning shoes."

Narrative notes are often used to document communication between team members and to record the results of team meetings, family conferences, home programs, and equipment assessments. As with all documentation, narrative notes should be grammatically correct, accurate, well organized, and concise and should reflect the clinical reasoning of the practitioner to support reimbursement of therapy services. Rambling, lengthy, and poorly organized notes that do not convey the clinical reasoning of the practitioner or identify the skilled service provided can jeopardize authorization for future services and reimbursement.

Reimbursement Requirements

Much of the documentation that takes place in clinical practice is driven by reimbursement requirements. The clinical record should supply sufficient evidence to support the need for occupational therapy intervention, including a statement about the client's baseline level of performance, prior level of function, objective and subjective information from assessments appropriate for the client age and diagnosis, clear and measurable short- and long-term objectives, and a detailed plan of treatment.

Documentation must be legible, relevant, and sufficient to justify the services billed (Centers for Medicare and Medicaid Services [CMS], 2009). Each of the many payer sources for occupational therapy services has specific requirements and standards for documentation. Medicare, the national insurance program for those ages 65 years or older, people ages 65 or younger with certain disabilities, and those with end-stage renal disease, sets national standards for documentation that other payer sources frequently follow when establishing documentation policies. Medicare outlines detailed documentation requirements for coverage of payment of occupational therapy services that identify the minimal expectations for documentation (CMS, 2009).

Documentation must clearly support that the services provided meet the requirements for medical necessity; that they are skilled, rehabilitative services provided by clinicians with the approval of a physician; and that they are safe and effective in promoting the rehabilitation of function. *Skilled services* are those that have a level of inherent complexity that requires the expertise, knowledge, clinical judgment, decision making, and abilities of an occupational therapy practitioner who has been trained to provide these services. These skills may be documented in the clinician's descriptions of his or her skilled intervention. Box 13.3 lists terminology used to describe skilled and unskilled occupational therapy services. Examples of skilled services include the following:

- The practitioner *assesses* the client's needs or progress and makes corresponding changes to the treatment program.
- The practitioner *determines* approaches or interventions to promote client safety. For example, a client with recent cardiac surgery requires close monitoring of heart rate and oxygen saturation levels during engagement in ADLs to determine safe levels of participation.
- The practitioner *instructs* a client in compensatory strategies. For example, a client learning techniques to achieve a safe swallow requires the skilled services of an occupational therapy practitioner to assess vocal quality, breathing, and changes in lung sounds that might indicate aspiration. Once the client is safe and independent in using the

BOX 13.3.
TERMINOLOGY INDICATING SKILLED VS. UNSKILLED SERVICES

Terminology Indicating Skilled Services	Terminology Indicating Unskilled Services
Adapt	Help
Analyze	Maintain
Assess	Monitor
Design	Observe
Determine	Practice
Develop	Watch
Establish	
Fabricate	
Facilitate	
Inhibit	
Instruct in (for example)	
• Compensatory strategies	
• Energy conservation techniques	
• Pursed lip breathing	
• Hemiplegic dressing techniques	
• Adaptive equipment	
• Coping strategies	
Interpret	
Modify	

compensatory techniques, the skills of the practitioner are no longer required, and further therapy would not be covered for this client unless the goals were modified.

Documentation of skilled services consists of a description of the activity, task, or modality, including a description of the therapeutic rationale underlying the activity, task, or modality choice. Documentation should also identify the variables that influenced the client's condition and identify the factors that influenced the practitioner's decision to recommend services (CMS, 2009). Complicating factors that affect the severity of the client's condition (e.g., medical, mental, age, time since onset, stability of symptoms) should also be identified in the client's record.

Legal and Ethical Concerns

Documentation is a permanent record of what occurred with the client and as such is a legal document. Anything written must be able to withstand a legal review should the need arise. It is the practitioner's responsibility to know what information is necessary to include in the client record for the specific practice setting and reimbursement intermediary.

All documentation must be accurate, complete, and based on firsthand knowledge of what occurred. Principle 6, Veracity, of the *Occupational Therapy Code of Ethics and Ethics Standards (2010)* (Code and Ethics Standards; AOTA, 2010) notes the following:

> By entering into a relationship in care or research, the recipient of service or research participant enters into a contract that includes a right to truthful information. . . . In addition, transmission of information is incomplete without also ensuring that the recipient or participant understands the information provided. (p. S23)

Principles 6B and 6D state that occupational therapy personnel shall "refrain from using or participating in any form of communication that contains false, fraudulent, deceptive, misleading, or unfair statements or claims" and "ensure that documentation for reimbursement purposes is done in accordance with applicable laws, guidelines, and regulations" (p. S24).

The occupational therapy practitioner is ethically and legally responsible for maintaining client confidentiality when communicating about the client in a written format. Principle 3H of the Code and Ethics Standards speaks to client confidentiality: "Occupational therapy personnel shall maintain the confidentiality of all verbal, written, electronic, augmentative, and nonverbal communications, including compliance with HIPAA regulations" (p. S21). *HIPAA* refers to the privacy sections of the Health Insurance Portability and Accountability Act of 1996 (P.L. 104–191), which protect consumers against breaches of confidentiality in medical settings.

The privacy standards were enacted in 2003 and regulate the use and disclosure of certain client information, called *protected health information (PHI)*, by health care providers, including occupational therapy practitioners. PHI includes any information that concerns health status or health care provision or that is related to a past, present, or future physical or mental health condition. This rule stipulates that the disclosure of PHI must be kept to the minimum necessary for health care professionals to carry out the purpose for which they are disclosing the information. HIPAA also gives clients the right of access to their medical records. In addition, the law requires that all personnel involved with client information at any level be trained in HIPAA policies and procedures and understand their implications specific to the work setting. The regulation applies to all written, verbal, and electronic communication, and violations are subject to criminal or civil sanctions (Fremgen, 2009).

Occupational therapy practitioners have a responsibility to protect confidential information from unauthorized access, use, or disclosure (Meyer & Schiff, 2004). This documentation cannot be disposed of in the regular trash; it must be shredded. Information cannot be shared with family members or others not directly involved with the care of the client unless the client provides written permission. Unauthorized people should never be allowed to view or have copies of client reports.

Issues in Electronic Documentation

Electronic documentation is becoming the norm in many practice settings, particularly in acute hospital and outpatient settings. Computerized documentation can increase practitioners' efficiency, resulting in increased productivity. Templates for evaluation, intervention, and outcome data can be developed to meet the specific needs of the practice setting and documentation requirements set by payer sources and accreditation agencies. Pull-down menus reduce the need for narrative entries and decrease the time spent in deciding on the appropriate terminology to use. Electronic information is readily available to all members of the health care team, which facilitates the exchange of key client information to enhance client care. In general, computerized documentation has been effective in increasing productivity by reducing the amount of time spent writing and is likely to become the preferred method of documentation.

Special care is required to preserve confidentiality in electronic documentation; staff should not share login pass codes, and they should always log off the computer after completing data entry. Practitioners must also take care to ensure that client privacy is maintained when entering information in a computer located in a public area such as a nursing station.

Users of electronic documentation must guard against several potential problems, however. Some practitioners may require additional time to grow accustomed to the technology used in computerized medical records. Practitioners may have to wait for a computer to become available to input their data; some settings alleviate this problem by providing handheld computers that practitioners can carry from client to client. Some electronic templates and forms restrict the information practitioners may enter, perhaps preventing them from documenting the results of therapy in the manner they feel is most appropriate.

Special care is required to preserve confidentiality in electronic documentation; staff should not share login pass codes, and they should always log off the computer after completing data entry. Practitioners must also take care to ensure that client privacy is maintained when entering information in a computer located in a public area such as a nursing station.

Writing Appropriate Documentation

Documentation is an important and necessary part of the occupational therapy process. Writing about what we do with our clients, why we do it, and what the outcomes of our interventions are helps explain the purpose of occupational therapy and provides evidence of its efficacy. Well-written documentation can provide valuable data for research and can contribute to the body of information necessary to support evidence-based practice. Skill in documenting the occupational therapy process helps occupational therapy practitioners accurately convey information about the client to others, ensures reimbursement of services and coverage of future services for clients, and provides ongoing proof of the value of occupational therapy intervention.

REFERENCES

American Occupational Therapy Association. (2008a). Guidelines for documentation of occupational therapy. *American Journal of Occupational Therapy, 62,* 684–690. doi:10.5014/ajot.62.6.684

American Occupational Therapy Association. (2008b). Occupational therapy practice framework: Domain and process (2nd ed.). *American Journal of Occupational Therapy, 62,* 625–683. doi:10.5014/ajot.62.6.625

American Occupational Therapy Association. (2010). Occupational therapy code of ethics and ethics standards (2010). *American Journal of Occupational Therapy, 64*(6 Suppl.), S17–S26. doi:10.5014/ajot.2010.64S17

Borcherding, S. (2005). *Documentation manual for writing SOAP notes in occupational therapy.* Thorofare, NJ: Slack.

Brennan, C., & Robinson, M. (2006). Documentation: Getting it right to avoid Medicare denials. *OT Practice, 11*(14), 10–15.

Centers for Medicare and Medicaid Services. (2009). *Medicare benefit policy manual: Chapter 15—Covered medical and other health services.* Retrieved from http://www.cms.gov/manuals/Downloads/bp102c15.pdf

Conrad, J. (2000). *Lord Jim quotes.* Calgary, Alberta, Canada: Broadview Press.

Fremgen, B. (2009). *Medical law and ethics* (3rd ed.). Upper Saddle River, NJ: Prentice Hall.

Health Insurance Portability and Accountability Act of 1996 (HIPAA), Pub. L. 104–191, 110 Stat. 1936. Retrieved from: http://www.cms.gov/Regulations-and-Guidance/HIPAA-Administrative-Simplification/HIPAAGenInfo/Downloads/HIPAALaw.pdf

Jackson, L. (Ed.). (2007). *Occupational therapy services for children and youth under IDEA* (3rd ed.). Bethesda, MD: AOTA Press.

Kettenbach, G. (2004). *Writing SOAP notes* (3rd ed.). Philadelphia: F. A. Davis.

Meyer, M., & Schiff, M. (2004). *HIPAA: The questions you didn't know to ask.* Upper Saddle River, NJ: Pearson/Prentice Hall.

Online Writing Laboratory at Purdue University. (2010). *Active versus passive voice.* Retrieved from http://owl.english.purdue.edu/owl/resource/539/02/

Sames, K. (2010). *Documenting occupational therapy practice* (2nd ed.). Upper Saddle River, NJ: Prentice Hall.

Schell, B. (2009). Clinical reasoning: The basis of practice. In E. Crepeau, E. Cohn, & B. Schell (Eds.), *Willard and Spackman's occupational therapy* (11th ed., pp. 314–327). Philadelphia: Lippincott Williams & Wilkins.

Smith, J. (2013). Documentation of occupational therapy services. In H. McHugh Pendleton & W. Schultz-Krohn (Eds.), *Pedretti's occupational therapy: Practice skills for physical dysfunction* (7th ed., pp. 117–139). St. Louis, MO: Elsevier Mosby.

Weed, L. (1971). *Medical records, medical education and patient care.* Chicago: Year Book Medical Publishers.

Writing for Your Career and for Payment

CHRISTINA A. DAVIS

The future of publishing is about having connections to readers and the knowledge of what those readers want.

—SETH GODIN (N.D.)

At some point in their careers, occupational therapy and other health care writers have collected a respectable number of *clips* (i.e., samples of writing such as magazine articles, news items, blogs) or research articles. Usually this coincides with writers reaching a point of expertise in their chosen profession, but sometimes it occurs earlier in a career, especially for entrepreneurs. Even though it is important to support one's profession—and one's career—by contributing to the knowledge base, it is equally important that skilled writers be compensated for sharing what they know.

This chapter shares a publishing professional's insights on navigating the world of publishing for payment, including finding the perfect partner, negotiating a contract, submitting a manuscript, handling rejection, and understanding the production process. Because the business models of content delivery are changing rapidly, the information provided is more general than specific to a particular type of publication or publisher and can apply to most print or electronic nonperiodical works (e.g., books, assessments).

Developing Ideas for Publications

Many writers have personal reasons for wanting to publish, whether reaching a career milestone, contributing to their curriculum vitae to secure a new position or tenure, or altruism. Within those motivations, writers may have new ideas or new approaches to information already published, including introducing more current evidence, using the latest technologies, or responding to today's realities. In addition, writers may notice that few products exist on an important topic, the views of their profession have not been included in a well-cited existing work, or the views of other professions would complement those of their own. Whatever the reason for wanting to publish, a publisher somewhere is likely interested in those ideas.

Finding a Publisher

Writers have several avenues to pursue in finding a publisher and can use the Internet to find the best fit for their work. In determining if a publisher is right for a project, writers can identify product niche and marketing style by seeing other products offered and how they are being sold. Web sites often host instructions for authors or list the latest topics of interest.

COMMERCIAL PUBLISHERS

Commercial publishers are often international corporations that usually produce a wide variety of books for a particular audience. *Trade publishers,* whose works are likely to appear in a local community bookstore, produce information for the general public—in health care, topics such as self-help, parenting, or health promotion. *STM publishers* (i.e., science, technical, medical), whose works are more likely to appear in a campus bookstore or university library, produce textbooks and similarly referenced works.

Commercial publishers usually have a large, often international, marketing reach, which could lead to more sales—and thus more royalties—for authors, as well as larger staffs who can produce much information in a short time. However, many commercial publishers are driven by tighter profit margins and so are ending advances or stipends to authors or subtracting production costs (e.g., proofreading, indexing) from those payments. This is particularly true in today's marketplace, as many of these publishers have exposure to declining real estate markets in the United States or to decreasing sales around the world in the wake of a global economic downturn.

NONPROFIT PUBLISHERS

Nonprofit publishers can be attached to a professional or trade association or to a nonprofit group and have a more defined audience for their work. Sometimes these publishers can produce a less profitable work because it fits with their mission, and they may have staff who are knowledgeable or expert on a particular topic. However, nonprofit publishers can have small staffs, tight budgets, and political considerations that can affect what and how often they publish.

SELF-PUBLISHING

Self-publishing, which has become more commonplace given new digital content development and delivery technologies, can be an option for entrepreneurial writers who are also strong self-promoters—and who have space to store printed inventory. Self-publishing companies include Amazon, Lulu, and BookSurge (it is beyond the scope of this chapter to discuss self-publishing in detail).

Although in theory this type of publishing seems accessible, authors must follow all quality control steps in production (e.g., securing proofreading, a professional design, a bar code, an ISBN number) to ensure product placement by bookstores or other distributors. Moreover, authors can be at the mercy of printers and other suppliers whose business rules may favor large publishers and not individual authors. For example, some online publishers and resellers are taking at least a 30% cut of a publication's profit and are discounting prices further, reducing the author's profit. Some printers are requiring that authors produce larger print runs than they can sell in a reasonable amount of time. Authors should fully understand contracts, business models, and payments before choosing a self-publishing partner.

> **Authors should fully understand contracts, business models, and payments before choosing a self-publishing partner.**

Understanding What Publishers Want

The Internet has made it much easier for aspiring authors to determine what publishers want to publish, either by reading the posted author guidelines or lists of preferred topics or by viewing the types of publications offered. Many publishers no longer read unsolicited manuscripts, so be sure to find the correct person to whom to send your work, and obtain permission to do so. Seek out staff with the titles "acquisitions editor" or "acquisitions associate." If those are not listed, look for a publishing or marketing "director" or "manager." Sending a proposal to a chief executive, however, is likely to cause a delay in the review of your work, because he or she is often involved in the business of acquiring other companies or product lines versus acquiring single titles.

BOX 14.1.

SAMPLE PROPOSAL AND MARKETING QUESTIONNAIRE ITEMS

Potential Items Needed for Submission

1. *Abstract (250 words or fewer):* Summary of the scope, purpose, and major points of the work
2. *Outline and contributors list:* Chapter outline, with key topics discussed in each, and details on potential contributors; planned page length and proposed formats for publication
3. *Sample chapter:* May be requested if publication is complete or to review writing style of new author
4. *Author background:* CV or résumé and one to two paragraphs about professional background and credentials
5. *Completed proposal form or marketing questionnaire or both.*

Potential Questions Asked in the Proposal Form

1. *Vision and goals:* Why do you want to publish this work? What will the work accomplish? What are the strengths and weaknesses of the work?
2. *Status:* What is the present status of the manuscript? Outline and sample chapter complete? Draft complete or near completion? What is your availability to complete the work?
3. *Format:* What is the proposed format of the work? What are the graphic or display needs of the work (e.g., photography, illustrations, figures, tables, case

If you are asked to complete a proposal form or marketing questionnaire, complete them in their entirety. In general, theses and dissertations do not make good book proposals, assessments require published research showing their clinical efficacy, and "everyone" is not a good response to the question "Who is the market for this work?"

MARKETABILITY OF IDEA

In making a decision on whether to publish a work, publishers try to determine audience type and size. Proposals from writers written in accessible (i.e., jargon-free) and concise language, indicating a well-defined idea and market, are likely to make it past the automated rejection e-mail. See Box 14.1 for sample questions on book proposal forms and marketing

---

BOX 14.1.

SAMPLE PROPOSAL AND MARKETING QUESTIONNAIRE ITEMS *(cont.)*

    examples, videos)? Are there parts of the work from other sources that will require permission to use?

4. *Publisher fit:* Why have you chosen [publisher] to publish the work? Has another publisher considered and declined to publish the work? Is another publisher presently considering the work?

5. *Reviewers:* Who are a few unbiased scholars in your field who have the expertise to review the work?

Potential Questions Asked in the Marketing Questionnaire

1. *Market size:* What is the potential market size? Where is the potential market (e.g., United States or international)?

2. *Target audience:* Who is the work's target audience? Practitioners? Students? Consumers? Is this a core or supplemental work?

3. *Competition:* What titles on the same topic compete with your work? How does your work differ from those titles?

4. *Promotion:* How do you think the work should be promoted? How will *you* promote the work? Have you had experience being interviewed or appearing on camera? Do you use social media?

5. *Motivation:* How can we motivate your target audience to buy the work now? In the future?

questionnaires, and be prepared to address these and similar questions when talking with publishing staff or deciding if you should self-publish.

Competition to the proposal is considered very carefully. Publishers see and talk to one another at various sales venues and publishing events, so staff generally know what is proposed or currently on the market. Saying that a work has no competition when it clearly does tells the publisher that a writer does not know the field very well (and in STM publishing, does not keep current in the relevant research), and so he or she is likely to produce an identical or derivative work with nothing new to offer readers. Even if a proposal has competition, a publisher is likely to take it on if the author has, for example, proposed a novel approach or introduced dynamic elements such as professionally produced videos.

AUTHOR REPUTATION

Publishers make decisions on the basis of author or editor name and reputation, commitment to the project, and expectations. Being a leader in the field, having the ability to stay on schedule, and assisting with marketing—which is evidenced in how well an author completes the marketing questionnaire—work in an author's favor.

However, in today's economic climate of finite resources and funding, no matter how important an author appears to be, if he or she complains about the time to make or outcome of the publishing decision, dismisses the instructions given to modify the work prior to acceptance, has plagiarized other works, or is generally rude or condescending to staff, a publisher is likely to reject the proposal (see also Chapter 5 in this volume for other items that publishers wish authors knew).

PUBLISHER RESOURCES

Publisher resources include editorial and marketing staff, platforms to deliver content in multiple formats, inventory and accounting systems, and the ability to resell content. Most publishers have decreased the number and types of staff in the past few years, and some have replaced in-house staff with freelance contractors or consultants. Many publishers also have experienced conflict between professional versus financial responsibility, especially to various stakeholders (e.g., shareholders, boards), and have cut back on the amount of, or passed on to the authors the costs of, quality control processes such as design, editing and proofreading, indexing, and reuse of nonoriginal materials. Therefore, publishers are seeking proposals that seem to require the least amount of effort to build quality content.

In addition, publishers are looking for opportunities for subsidiary rights and repackaging (i.e., additional places to sell content). These include translations, placement with aggregators such as EBSCO or OVID, and selling by piece (i.e., selling individual chapters as well as entire books).

Knowing What to Ask

While publishers are asking authors what they have to offer, authors should be asking—politely—what publishers can provide to them.

First, determine personal fit with a publisher. Is the publisher in the same marketplace as your proposed product? Are staff committed to your ideas or profession? Are business practices in line with your views on the environment, accessibility, or politics? Do staff personalities work with yours?

Second, ask about editorial and marketing resources. Although they may not know with which staff person an author would be working, publishers can explain their processes for content development, production, and marketing. Smaller publishers usually provide more personalized attention, and larger publishers usually move more quickly toward a final product.

Third, and only after establishing a relationship, ask about contracts and royalties (asking earlier tells the publisher that you are more interested in payment than in producing the work). Contract templates vary, as does a publisher's flexibility in altering standard wording, which likely has been vetted through attorneys. Contracts cover copyright ownership, author or publisher reuse of information (i.e., noncompete clauses), payments, deadlines, and scope of work.

There is varying flexibility in negotiating contracts. More-established authors are likely to receive a higher payment or larger percentage of royalties. A core text is likely to sell more than a supplemental text (i.e., larger market), and so the contracts for these should feature better payment terms. However, both royalties and payments have been shrinking, so it is

> **Both royalties and payments have been shrinking, so it is likely that even responsible authors of great products could see their terms change between editions.**

likely that even responsible authors of great products could see their terms change between editions. Thus, it is important to know whether the payment is in line with the industry standard.

Authors can expect reasonable timelines, usually negotiated with the author's schedule in mind. Look for competitive payments, and ask about possible deductions from the stipend or advance for production costs or late delivery of the manuscript. Determine if the publisher will be reselling the content and if you will be paid if they do; many publishers do this but generate addenda to contracts only after an agreement is in place with a reseller.

Copyright ownership and noncompete clauses are places where both sides can find themselves at an impasse (see Chapter 6 in this volume). STM publishers generally will hold copyright, as they are highly likely to resell work. An exception to this is for assessments, where it can be commonplace to allow the author to hold the rights—and responsibilities of policing the work as well as selling rights. This occurs often because assessments need to be recalibrated for changes in country or population served, and the authors are best equipped to do this.

Noncompete clauses cannot be removed from contracts but usually can be refined to cover an author's concerns. The standard language is rather strong, but most publishers will accommodate changes to clarify that reusing the information for teaching or presenting, as well as to publish research articles, for example, are allowed.

Handling Rejection

Knowing that a publisher is not rejecting you personally but just one of your ideas can help authors reorganize thoughts to resubmit or to find another publisher. Many publishers can make suggestions for a better home for the work (unless an author was discourteous during the review process; even with the sometimes fierce rivalries that exists among publishers, few publishing staff would risk their reputations by deliberately sending someone unsuitable to their competitors—their potential next employers).

Publishers may also encourage authors to resubmit to them later, when, for example, an emerging practice area has more research supporting its efficacy or the business climate seems better suited to support the work. Unless the work is completely unsuitable (such as a nursing work submitted to an occupational therapy publisher), the publisher has invested some time researching an author's background and imagining the proposal in its line for products and would likely be interested in that author for future endeavors.

Two exceptions to this are children's books and products with strong religious content. The marketplace is full of specialized children's book publishers (e.g., Woodbine House, Autism Asperger Publishing), and submitting a children's book to, for example, an STM publisher is not appropriate. Works with strong religious content, particularly espousing the view of a particular religion over all others, are very likely to be rejected out of hand and fit better with a religion publisher, from which there are many to choose, even in the health care marketplace.

Also, it is becoming more common for publishers to cancel contracts, either for author nonperformance or, more likely, because of changing business conditions (e.g., publisher is purchased by another publisher, publication topic no longer part of publisher's line) in the middle of production. If for the latter reason, authors usually can keep whatever has been paid to them so far in the publication process and can ask the publisher for a letter returning the rights as well as a reference to use when shopping the work to another publisher.

Navigating Production

Publishers manage production according to their unique staffing availability and business processes. The following is a general guide to what occurs and authors' roles in this process.

PREPUBLICATION MARKETING

During prepublication marketing, which begins before the manuscript is due from the author to the publisher, titles are chosen, cover and interior designs are developed (these days, usually designed with Internet sales and digital delivery in mind). Once a manuscript has been reviewed by the publisher, staff determine final costs for production and then project prices for the work.

In all of these processes, publishers will seek the input of authors, but the publisher almost always has the last word. Titles are chosen to accurately reflect content and to enhance *discoverability,* that is, to help readers who do not know the title of the work find the work. Most publishers are well versed in the taxonomy of the professions they represent and have at least a decade of experience posting titles to Amazon.com or their own online sales platforms and so understand the marketplace and which key words to use.

As part of the publishing partnership, authors can let the publisher know if there are colors or images that they dislike and will usually see cover "comps" (i.e., samples) as a courtesy. However, unless the treatment is an actual violation of, for example, a religious edict of the author, the cover design is final.

PEER REVIEW AND DEVELOPMENTAL (OR COPY) EDITING

Most STM publishers use peer review (i.e., review by a qualified professional or educator in the same profession) to make certain that all pertinent topics and, if appropriate, points of view have been covered in a manuscript. Authors are expected to submit names of impartial reviewers in their fields, and publishers also maintain a core group of internal and external reviewers.

At the same time, developmental editors begin work to ensure readability. Developmental editors see the "big picture" of a work and look for accuracy in facts, math, or statistics; amount of documentation or citation; completeness of ideas; and logical organization.

Most authors will likely receive comments from peer reviewers and developmental editors; it is a rare manuscript that needs no revisions. Authors must follow the instructions and resubmit by the deadline given or explain to the publisher why they disagree with the requested changes. The publisher may or may not require the revisions to be made, but if it does want the work completed and the author does not complete it in a timely manner, the publisher will put the work on hold or cancel the contract, before additional funds are spent on the project.

COPYEDITING

Once any major revisions are made, manuscripts are edited in a word-processing program, showing changes or not, and often are passed through an automated redacting program. With input from the author, the publisher gives copy editors a checklist of items for correcting—in addition to grammar, consistency, organization, or people-first language—and queries for unclear or missing items, as well as instructions to follow a particular style (see Chapter 4 in this volume for more information on grammar, Chapter 7 for more information on style). The publisher instructs the editor on the level of editing required—identified in peer review or by the publisher as light, medium, or heavy.

After copyediting is completed, the author carefully reviews the marked-up manuscript, resolves any queries, and returns the manuscript by the deadline. Authors should expect a high-quality, consistent editing job. If any disagreements arise, it is likely that the author will prevail if the problem is in the content and the publisher will prevail if the problem is in the style.

TYPESETTING AND FILE MAINTENANCE

Once a manuscript has been edited and reviewed, it is ready for typesetting, which is running the text into the interior design template using a program such as InDesign. This process can take a few days to a few weeks, depending on the size of the work. For publishers who are producing digital works, the file may also be saved as XML or HTML5.

It is becoming more common for authors to encounter information technology professionals during production, especially with digital publications (University of Chicago Press, 2010). Publishers may ask authors to develop more dynamic, "show-me" elements such as videos, reader test questions or tasks to complete, and instructor guides for their publications. Authors should feel free to ask about any elements they do not understand but should know that publishers may not proceed with the work if these items are not developed in a timely and affordable way. Many publishers have access to, for example, video production but may need authors to write scripts.

PROOFREADING AND INDEXING

Authors usually have the opportunity to review page proofs created in these formats and will be asked to make only minor corrections on a short deadline. The proofs may show instances of computer coding or other items that will be invisible once the files are finalized.

While the author is reviewing the proofs, a professional proofreader will be looking as well for editorial or formatting errors. Both the author and proofreader may be asked to mark corrections directly on a PDF using electronic marking tools. However, some publishers have removed the proofreading step

> **Some publishers have removed the proofreading step from production to save money and so may rely on authors alone to find mistakes.**

from production to save money and so may rely on authors alone to find mistakes.

During this time an indexer or the author will create an index for the print version of the book, using headings and key words as a guide. It is important to make as few corrections as possible in reviewing proofs to avoid shifting text and causing mistakes in the index.

Editors of multiauthored works are expected to reconcile the proofs of all authors into one set and return it to the publisher.

PRINTING AND MANUFACTURING

Once all corrections are in, the typesetter prepares and checks electronic text and cover files for the printer or digital delivery platform. The publisher usually reviews at least portions of the work one final time (e.g., bluelines), and then the work is manufactured or loaded on the digital platform. The finished print product is delivered to a fulfillment center or warehouse for distribution. The entire process can take from mere days to months depending on the complexity of the product.

FULFILLMENT AND POSTPUBLICATION MARKETING

The distribution center answers questions about products from script prepared from the marketing questionnaire. Center staff process and ship orders, as well as grant access to e-book files. The publisher's order inventory and accounting systems track sales and other information, which are used to calculate royalties. Once a product is completed, authors are generally paid the remainder of their stipend or advance.

At this point, authors can help the publisher market the product by encouraging customers to purchase it through reader reviews on social media sites or by promoting or selling the book at any meetings or events they attend.

REVISIONS AND CANCELLATIONS

Publishers seek revisions for successful products—those that have sold well and have received favorable reviews. Revisions previously occurred every 5 to 7 years but now happen more quickly, especially in STM publishing, as the latest research often can make the statements in a work outdated.

Staff will determine whether a work is eligible for revision or if it will go "out of print" (i.e., be cancelled). Authors almost always gain the rights to a work that a publisher has declined to revise and may be offered a chance to purchase the remaining inventory before it is destroyed or recycled.

For revisions, authors can ask trusted colleagues for their ideas or use social media to generate feedback. The publisher will solicit feedback as well from previous purchasers and, for textbooks, from educators who have adopted the work.

In digital publishing, revisions can be ongoing, with authors asked to remain attached to the project to answer reader questions, update links, and make reference lists more current.

It is not unusual for a publisher to plan a revision with an author even before issuing the first royalty payment, especially if the changes in the field are somewhat predictable (e.g., the federal government will release new data at predetermined times, a large research project on the subject is nearing completion). In addition, a publisher or author may have uncovered a new topic of interest during production of the previous project and, if the existing arrangement has been successful, may pursue a contract with an author for new work.

For an author who has performed well, a publisher may be willing to wait for him or her to complete other projects—even those with competing publishers—and will sign an "intent to contract" or a memorandum of understanding to secure a future place in the author's schedule for the revision or new product.

Collecting Your Payment

Many authors receive stipends or advances, paid throughout the content development process, as well as royalties, often paid twice a year on a predetermined schedule, usually after inventory has been counted or at the end of a fiscal or calendar year. Authors are usually asked to complete documents such as W-9s and banking electronic transfer forms before their first stipend or royalties are paid (these documents often are part of the contract). For authors who have had difficulties with the Internal Revenue Service, the government does garnish royalties and stipends to cover outstanding tax liabilities.

Understanding the Publishing Relationship

Many opportunities exist for authors to receive payment for their work that include working with a publisher or self-publishing. When working with a publisher, authors should remember that, although their relationship is a partnership, each has different responsibilities. Publishers make a substantial investment in developing an author's content and want authors to be successful. Authors have an opportunity to receive payment and add to their career achievements and also want to be successful. Understanding what both parties want from the relationship can help authors find the right publishing fit and build long-term contracts that benefit both partners.

REFERENCES

Godin, S. (n.d.). *Publishing.* Available online at http://www.brainyquote.com/quotes/keywords/publishing_3.html

University of Chicago Press. (2010). Production and digital technology. In *The Chicago manual of style: The essential guide for writers, editors, and publishers* (16th ed., pp. 861–890). Chicago: Author.

Writing and Communicating in the New Media

PART IV

Presentations: Overcoming a Fear Worse Than Death

RONDALYN V. WHITNEY, PhD, OT/L

Be who you are and say what you feel because "those who mind don't matter and those who matter don't mind."
—BERNARD BARUCH (AS CITED IN CERF, 1948, P. 249)

*P*ublic speaking. Do those words cause your heart to accelerate, your mouth to get dry, or your hands to sweat? Or are you thinking about opportunities to share your knowledge with others, feeling that to do so is a professional responsibility? Delivering presentations to others is an important act of advocacy, an example of activism. Your knowledge can benefit others' practice only if you disseminate that knowledge.

As occupational therapists, we must communicate our professional ideas, research outcomes, and understanding of human wellness, quality of life, and the benefits of occupation, and we must do so outside our own small circles of fellow practitioners. The ability to give an effective presentation, like any other skill, is honed through experience and perseverance. Speakers cultivate the characteristics highly valued by audiences: credibility and knowledge, enthusiasm for the topic, and the ability to connect with the audience. These skills are within the well-used toolkit of any occupational therapist, teacher, or clinician.

BOX 15.1.
SIX STEPS TO BECOMING A SUCCESSFUL PRESENTER

- Step 1. Select a topic.
- Step 2. Research your topic.
- Step 3. Refine your content.
- Step 4. Prepare yourself.
- Step 5. Don't be a bore.
- Step 6. Seize opportunities to present.

Writer Anaïs Nin said, "Life shrinks or expands in proportion to one's courage." I would add that behind most courageous acts is a person prepared to take action. You may feel a little (or a lot) nervous about presenting in front of an audience. You can, however, rise to the occasion with a passion for your topic, some preparation, and strategies for calming your butterflies.

This chapter is intended to bolster your audacity to prepare and deliver an interesting and informative presentation. After a discussion of the many reasons to present, I outline six steps you can take to become a successful presenter (Box 15.1).

Reasons to Present

If you are not already an expert on a specific topic, preparation of a presentation might make you one! You will have the chance to gather the newest findings, tap the experts, and even influence the audience's attitudes about a topic. Each time you present, you face down your anxiety, develop your skills, and feel more comfortable when you present the next time. You might have to make a professional presentation for career advancement purposes; to ready your staff for a new type of equipment, protocol, research method, or technology; or to address an identified need in the community. If you are comfortable with preparing a presentation, you can volunteer more easily, you may have more liberty in selecting your subject matter, and you will be recognized for your independence and willingness to support your organization.

For example, Martha was an occupational therapist providing intervention for students in a public school, and she often provided a home program to improve hand function as a support for better handwriting. The school principal asked Martha to present at the annual back-to-school parent training as part of their welcome event. Martha knew how to help students develop better hand function, but in preparing for the presentation, she found new research on the evidence supporting better outcomes for handwriting in students with autism, attention deficit hyperactivity disorder, and typically developing children. She increased her expertise as she added the evidence to her clinical knowledge and crafted a presentation that translated the latest research into practical application for the audience of families and teachers. She arranged for several of her students to join her and demonstrate her practice techniques. She also distributed handouts of some of the great resources she had downloaded from the American Occupational Therapy Association (AOTA).

Becoming a Successful Presenter

STEP 1. SELECT A TOPIC

The first step in developing a presentation is to select a topic. Draw from your area of expertise. A presentation is essentially a story you are sharing with your audience. Everyone has something they know well that would be of value to others in practice or personally. What are you an expert on? Perhaps you have cracked the code on fitting exercise into your schedule or have a way of getting healthy meals prepared for a family of six while working full-time. Perhaps you recently worked with a patient who had an unusual condition that inspired you to plan an innovative therapeutic technique. Maybe you recently researched a unique set of symptoms related to a rare disorder, learned about an innovative intervention, or worked with an interesting case and developed a case study. Maybe you read a book about motivation and would like to share what you discovered about intrinsic and extrinsic rewards. Maybe you have a personal story to share.

There is really only one rule to follow when choosing a topic: Pick a topic you are passionate about. Your natural enthusiasm will come across in your voice and your body language, and you will enjoy preparing for your presentation.

> There is really only one rule to follow when choosing a topic: Pick a topic you are passionate about.

Another way to identify a topic is to think the way you do when you conduct a needs assessment for a client: What problem does your audience have that your presentation can help them solve? Do they, for example, need to decrease documentation time? Improve the balance between work and home? Have an environmental face-lift to optimize employee and client morale? If you have a solution, people will want to hear it.

I once went to a presentation on scrapbooking for mothers of preemies. It was outstanding because the presenter was passionate (she was the mom of a preemie), she loved scrapbooking, and she was deeply committed to finding a way to provide a caring activity for mothers when, as she well knew, they were most in need of caring. I was moved and inspired and really felt how such a seemingly simple occupation could be so powerful.

When you've identified your topic, give it a catchy title. Instead of "How to Set Up a Facebook Account," consider "How Millennial Are You? Friends and Facebook."

STEP 2. RESEARCH YOUR TOPIC

Once you decide on the subject for your talk and have a catchy title, you need to explore what has already been said on the subject. It will take you some time to search, retrieve, and review the literature you find. Don't be surprised if you get lost in what you find; this is an area of interest for you, after all. Google Scholar (a search engine for scholarly literature) is a great place to start, and many libraries and journals now make full-text articles available online.

You can't expect to exhaust the literature using only open-access (i.e., free) journals, but online databases are increasingly being offered as a membership benefit through state occupational therapy professional associations. Of course, if you're an AOTA member, you have online access to articles from the *American Journal of Occupational Therapy, OT Practice,* and the Special Interest Section quarterly newsletters.

STEP 3. REFINE YOUR CONTENT

In refining the content of your presentation, begin by developing key points and learning objectives, and then develop a content outline that covers each point and objective.

Key Points
Identify 3 to 5 key points for your talk. I like to use an organizing framework such as the *Occupational Therapy Practice Framework: Domain and Process*

(AOTA, 2008) or other tools of the profession. For example, if you wanted to present on children with autism, you may wish to organize your paper around the performance skills affected (i.e., motor and praxis, sensory-perceptual, emotional-regulation, cognitive skills, communication, and social skills).

Learning Objectives

Learning objectives define what learners will know or be able to do after attending your presentation. Your learning objectives should flow from your key points.

In developing learning objectives (Mager, 1997) for your presentation, keep in mind the knowledge level of your audience—beginner, intermediate, or advanced—when deciding what new skills, knowledge, or attitudes you want learners to acquire. Bloom's (1956) taxonomy (see also Pohl, 2000) suggests framing learning objectives using the acronym SKA:

- *S*kills (What will learners be able to do after your presentation?),
- *K*nowledge (What will learners know?), and
- *A*ttitudes (How will your presentation change learners' opinions?).

Consider writing one learning objective for each skill, knowledge, and attitude component of your presentation. List your learning objectives in order from lower levels of challenge to more complex learning. For example, learning a protocol is less challenging than evaluating or creating a protocol. Bloom suggested that learners will, in order of increasing difficulty, know, comprehend, apply, analyze, evaluate/synthesize, and create. Your learning objectives should follow this gradation and use these verbs to indicate level of complexity. For example,

At the end of my presentation, learners will be able to [insert verb from Bloom's taxonomy, such as *know, explain, demonstrate, evaluate, analyze, create*] about [one key point of your topic].

- ***For a beginner audience, you might say***—*At the end of this presentation, learners will be able to recognize (know) the performance skills affected by the diagnosis of autism.*
- ***For an intermediate audience you might say***—*At the end of this presentation, learners will be able to apply three sensory strategies and evaluate effect on tabletop tasks.*

> In general, audiences highly value practical information and an outline that gives them a broad idea of what you will cover, the time you plan to allot to each area, and the resources they can follow up on when they get home.

- *For an advanced audience, you might say*—At the end of this presentation, learners will be able to evaluate performance skill deficits and create evidence-based treatment plans for children in Grades 1–5.

Good learning objectives are realistic and measurable, even if you do not intend to formally evaluate participants' achievement. Consider, however, using an informal evaluation technique such as asking your audience members to give a short report to demonstrate understanding, to take a before-and-after test to measure changes in opinion, or to work together in small groups to create a lesson plan of their own.

Content Outline

Once your main points and learning objectives are in order, write a detailed content outline containing the supporting information for your main points and learning objectives, keeping in mind your available time. In general, audiences highly value practical information and an outline that gives them a broad idea of what you will cover, the time you plan to allot to each area, and the resources they can follow up on when they get home.

For example, the introduction to a presentation about work-related stress and leisure could include facts and statistics, making the case for the importance of the suggested intervention, and a tangible/experiential example of what participants can do immediately upon the conclusion of the presentation. Provide an activity that will allow for an "ah-ha moment," and then make sure you provide time for questions and answers but have an alternate activity in hand if there are no questions (something you can either present or provide a handout for if you don't have time).

Therefore, your outline for a 1½-hour presentation might look like this:

I. Leisure as the antidote for work-related stress
   A. Introduction and definition (20 minutes)
      a. Work-related stress
      b. Leisure

    B. Scope and significance of the problem (20 minutes)
       a. Prevalence and risks of stress
       b. The decline of leisure
    C. Breakout activity (20 minutes)
       a. Rediscovering leisure interests using the Leisure Inventory
       b. Group discussion
    D. Health benefits from engaging in leisure pursuits (15 minutes)
    E. Question/answer and additional resources (15 minutes).

STEP 4. PREPARE YOURSELF

After developing a content outline, decide on a structure for your presentation that specifies which content you will discuss at what point. Most presentations you make will include the use of PowerPoint, and remembering some key points will make your slides and your presentation complement rather than compete against each other (Reynolds, 2010; Williams, 2009).

I like to borrow a technique from an artist I worked with: The eye finds 3 items more appealing than 2 and less overwhelming than 4. For a crowd-pleasing presentation, use the rule of 3: 1 point, 3 examples, break, then repeat. If your presentation is to last 2 hours, give three 20-minute presentations, allowing additional time for the introduction, activities, summary, and questions.

Guy Kawasaki (2005), an evangelist for Macintosh, developed the 10/20/30 rule for PowerPoint presentations. He said PowerPoint presentations are "quite simple: A PowerPoint presentation should have 10 slides, last no more than 20 minutes, and contain no font smaller than 30 points." A 2-hour presentation might be structured as follows:

1. Introduction and review of the learning objectives (10 minutes)
2. A quote or play on words (10 minutes)
3. Objective 1 (10 slides, 20 minutes)
4. Activity (10 minutes)
5. Objective 2 (10 slides, 20 minutes)
6. Activity (10 minutes)
7. Objective 3 (10 slides, 20 minutes)
8. Activity (10 minutes)
9. Summary and questions (10 minutes).

If you are presenting for longer than 2 hours, take an extended break after the first 2 hours or plan a small-group activity after 60 minutes, and repeat the steps in the structure until you are done. You should specify the time frame of your presentation in your introduction and include appropriate amounts of content to enable you to begin and end each segment on time. All speakers must respect time limitations, allowing the audience to keep their own schedules and commitments. When speakers run overtime, the audience may get restless, preoccupied, or even angry.

If you wait to present until you feel "completely comfortable" speaking in front of a crowd, you may never do it. Courage is not about not feeling afraid; courage is about acting even when you feel anxious or fearful. But how can you be prepared to still your butterflies?

First, remember that presenting is a learned skill. Start small and build up your muscle. Preparation and rehearsal will go a long way in decreasing your stress level. Practice in your mirror, practice with one or two good friends, learn the major points of your outline so you have a clear picture in your mind of where you are at each point of the presentation. When you are confident you know your topic, you will feel much more confident in front of an audience. Next, take some time to think about your style. Are you more comfortable presenting the facts? Do you like to have a dialogue with others? Are you funny? Capitalize on your strengths, and you'll feel more comfortable when you present your information.

Plan to start your presentation and each point with something catchy like a joke, a quote, a cartoon, an anecdote, a personal example, a video clip, or a short activity. Think about kicking off with a puzzle, a mystery, something with suspense. I once began a presentation on using sensory strategies in the classroom with a guessing game. I passed a box around and had the audience guess what was inside by using their senses—looking at it, shaking it and listening, lifting it up to guess its weight, and smelling it. I passed it around until everyone had a chance to use his or her own senses to learn about the box. Whoever guessed what was inside got to keep the prize.

Another attention-getter is to ask for volunteers throughout your presentation. For example, if you want to help your audience understand *proximity* (i.e., the appropriate social space in interactions with others), you may call up a volunteer and explain a concept to him or her while standing *way* too close. Consider providing a small reward for your helper, something that furthers your point. In this example, I might give the participant a measuring tape and then go on to explain that I show children how to measure the 3 feet of social space considered appropriate in the United States. When I present on therapeutic humor, I ask volunteers to share or participate in a joke and reward him or her with a rubber chicken, clown nose, or other comedy gag. Later in the presentation, when we work in small groups to develop personal humor kits, the gags serve as inspiration for the participants.

Consider leaving your audience with some food for thought. I often include a few slides at the end entitled "Additional Material for Your Toolkit" on which I list facts, goals, recipes, or other pertinent information for those who are interested. Consider a "Were you paying attention?" slide, on which you list five or six questions that reiterate and reinforce your overall objectives. You can toss a small treat or gift to those who answer these questions to encourage the group to respond. Or, as you conclude your presentation, return to your learning objectives and tell the audience, "Let's see if I met my objectives." Reread each one, waiting for the audience to affirm that you successfully met your objectives. Handouts are another way to indicate to your audience that you believe the topic is important and expect them to want further information. The audience will be impressed that you took the time and trouble to provide further resources.

STEP 5. DON'T BE A BORE

Successful speakers show they have a command of the materials they are presenting; they stay focused and show they are well prepared. Audiences respond positively to neat, well-groomed, stylish speakers, so do pay attention to your appearance. Audiences also respond favorably to speakers who are animated and interesting. If you have special characteristics or talents, such as a high energy level or the ability to draw quick sketches or tell humorous anecdotes, use those skills to engage your group.

Preparation and practice enhance presentations by increasing the effectiveness of the speaker. As you make more presentations, you will raise your comfort level, which audience members will see reflected in your speech patterns and nonverbal gestures. Be enthusiastic, and tell the group you are happy to be addressing them on this exciting topic. Audiences appreciate not only a credible and knowledgeable speaker but also one who is interesting and enthusiastic and has an easygoing manner. Finally, a sense of humor goes a long way to win an audience and add spark to the presentation. Table 15.1 lists common pitfalls in presenting and ways to avoid them.

TABLE 15.1. Common Pitfalls in Presenting to an Audience and Effective Solutions

Pitfall	Solution
Spending too much time fiddling with uncooperative technology	• Send someone out for tech support. • Have and implement a backup plan. If you know your materials, and your audience has a handout, you can proceed without the PowerPoint.
Reading from your slides	• Use a large (30-point) font, and display only the key points. • Prepare ahead of time by making notes about the specific points you want to make. • Present 3 lines of text on each slide, and practice the 3 points you wish to make about each of those key points. • Rely on the rule of 3: 1 point, 3 examples, break, then repeat.
Being interrupted by questions	• Announce your rule for questions: You can take them at the end, the middle, or throughout, but be firm. • Consider handing out index cards to larger groups and pausing after each 2-hour block to review and answer questions from the audience. • If you want a more interactive group, consider giving small prizes for good questions or comments.
Acknowledging typos and other errors in your written materials	• No one is perfect. Consider announcing up front that you have a prize for anyone who spots a typo on your slides and submits an index card pointing it out; award prizes at the end of your presentation. • If you know you have an error, admit the error, and state clearly the corrected version. Address a typo by saying something like, "Oh, a typo. I always have one, and look, I've found it early in the presentation!" Remember, the audience is on your side.
Starting or ending late	• Don't start late; it is disrespectful to those who arrived on time. Consider a compromise—use the first 10 minutes to provide informal or nonessential information or find out who is in the audience. • Don't run over—end on time. Offer to stay to answer questions, but after you formally dismiss the group.

Nothing is worse for an audience than watching a presenter spend 20 minutes fussing with technology—the audience came to hear you speak, not to see your slides. Have a backup plan for how to proceed in the event of a technology breakdown. And whatever you do, don't stand and read your slides; this is boring to the audience and suggests that you are unsure of yourself or your presentation.

> **Whatever you do, don't stand and read your slides; this is boring to the audience and suggests that you are unsure of yourself or your presentation.**

When you step up to the podium or in front of the audience, stand quietly for a minute, take a few deep breaths, smile, and look around at the friendly people who, after all, have come to hear what you have to say. And remember, you do have something to say, something, in fact, that you feel passionate about sharing.

And although it may seem obvious, don't forget to breathe, and breathe deeply, down into the lower lobes of your lungs. When you are anxious, you have a tendency to breathe in a shallow manner, resulting in less oxygen in your system and even hyperventilation. This will cause your vocal cords to overstretch and your voice to sound squeezed or strained, and you will feel out of breath. The less air you take in, the worse you feel, and the worse you feel, the less air you take in. Good breathing habits break this cycle.

If you regulate your breathing, your body will respond physiologically by relaxing. Breathing is underrated, but don't take it for granted! Stand up straight, and relax your shoulders. Breathe in through your nose to the count of 10, counting slowly, and exhale out of your mouth, again counting slowly to 10. Throughout your presentation, continue to take deep, calming breaths. Table 15.2 lists other symptoms of nervousness and suggests antidotes.

The ending of your presentation is as important as the beginning. As a speaker, never act as if you are relieved that the presentation is over. Remain upbeat, confident, and strong to the last word. When wrapping up the session, allow yourself a few minutes to emphasize and summarize salient points, highlights, or conclusions. This is also the time to identify your future projects and plans.

Volunteer to stay after the presentation to speak with participants who want further assistance or have other comments to make. You may want to say, "We're out of time, so I will end there. I know many of you need to [get back to work, go to your next session], but I'm happy to stick around if

TABLE 15.2. Symptoms of and Antidotes for Nervousness

Symptom	Antidote
Dry mouth	Have water or hot tea ready and take sips.
Trembling hands	Put your hands together, hold your own hand, or hold something heavy.
Knocking knees	Shift your weight, unlock your knees, or sit on a high stool for your presentation.
Shaking voice	Take a deep breath or two, or look at someone in the audience and smile.
Sweating	If you sweat, wear clothing that will not show perspiration, and then forget about it.
Fear of embarrassing yourself	Visualize success. Picture yourself walking up to the front of the room looking confident. Imagine yourself at the end, having delivered a successful presentation. Practice your key points over and over until you feel confident you are the expert on your topic!

anyone has questions or would like to speak with me further." If you need to clear the room because another speaker is waiting, suggest, "I'm happy to meet you outside and continue our conversation further." Audience members will appreciate your sensitivity to their time constraints, and those with additional questions will appreciate your availability.

Think about it: After all, what is the worst that can happen? Will the entire audience get up and walk out? Will they point and laugh? Will they fall asleep and snore? Will they throw tomatoes? You're most unlikely to experience any of these if you prepare and present something you're passionate about. Most audiences will, at the worst, just think you are poorly prepared.

When you are done with your presentation, take inventory. Use each experience to learn about yourself and grow as a speaker.

STEP 6. SEIZE OPPORTUNITIES TO PRESENT

Polished presenters buff their skills by constantly speaking. You can strengthen your abilities by presenting at local parent–teacher association meetings, local university or community college events, your state or national professional association's annual conference, and other public-speaking venues.

Small, familiar groups may be less threatening and more relaxed, and they are usually pleased to have speakers talk about health care and occupational science topics. Such groups usually do not have a formal mechanism to solicit speakers. You just contact someone who is responsible for the meeting agenda or the event and tell them about your talk, and they will let you know if they are interested and, if so, what steps you need to take next. For example, if you wish to present to your coworkers about an innovative technique, you might speak with your department chair to see if there will be some open time during an upcoming staff meeting you could use for your presentation.

Most professional organizations have annual conferences with both invited (paid) and selected (volunteer) speakers. The larger the organization, the more formal the process for soliciting speakers. Visit the Web site of organizations you think would be a good fit for your presentation, and watch for calls for papers that announce the theme of the conference, guidelines for the types of presentations they are looking for (e.g., workshops, roundtables, all-day institutes), and the deadline for submission. See Chapter 9 for more information on presenting at conferences.

Follow Your Passion to Present Successfully

The six steps presented in this chapter will help you feel more confident in preparing and presenting your ideas to an audience. If you follow your passions, you will be successful. When I see you at the front of the room, I will look forward to learning something new, developing a new skill, and being inspired by an idea about which you are passionate.

REFERENCES

American Occupational Therapy Association. (2008). Occupational therapy practice framework: Domain and process (2nd ed.). *American Journal of Occupational Therapy, 62*, 625–683. doi:10.5014/ajot.62.6.625

Bloom, B. S. (1956). *Taxonomy of educational objectives: Book 1. The cognitive domain.* New York: David McKay.

Cerf, B. (1948). *Shake well before using: A new collection of impressions and anecdotes mostly humorous.* New York: Simon & Schuster.

Kawasaki, G. (2005). *The 10/20/30 rule of PowerPoint.* Retrieved September 27, 2011, from http://blog.guykawasaki.com/2005/12/the_102030_rule.html#axzz1ZBa0b69V

Mager, R. F. (1997). *Preparing instructional objectives: A critical tool in the development of effective instruction.* Atlanta: Center for Effective Performance.

Pohl, M. (2000). *Learning to think, thinking to learn: Models and strategies to develop a classroom culture of thinking.* Cheltenham, Victoria, Australia: Hawker Brownlow.

Reynolds, G. (2010). *The naked presenter: Delivering powerful presentations with or without slides* (Voices That Matter series). Berkeley, CA: New Riders Press.

Williams, R. (2009). *The non-designer's presentation book.* Berkeley, CA: Peachpit Press.

Conducting Virtual Meetings: A New Form of Communication

BRENT BRAVEMAN, PhD, OTR/L, FAOTA

The first rule of any technology used in a business is that automation applied to an efficient operation will magnify the efficiency. The second is that automation applied to an inefficient operation will magnify the inefficiency.
—BILL GATES (N.D.)

In the past decade the use of social media Web sites and new communication and meeting platforms has exploded. As access to the Internet has become commonplace and wireless, we have the ability to interact with others around the globe in real time. We can view and edit documents simultaneously, hold "live meetings" in which large groups of people combine online viewing with a conference call, hold group chats, and see one another from our homes through video conferencing. In the span of a few decades—within the career lifespans of many of us—the virtual world has transformed how we interact and how we do business. This transformation has provided untold opportunities to share information and increase productivity.

The proliferation of virtual communication and meeting tools allows occupational therapy managers, educators, clinicians, and other practitioners a broader opportunity to communicate. Using these tools effectively requires the development of a unique set of communication skills. In addition, the rise of virtual communications, which are often absent the face-to-face interaction that allows us to read body and facial cues, tone of voice, and other contextual information, can be fraught with problems. This chapter explores the most common evolving virtual communication tools, how to make the most of them, and how to avoid the most common disruptive pitfalls.

Past and Present-Day Electronic Communication

Personal computers, the Internet, and other wireless and virtual communication mechanisms have transformed where and when we do business in just a few decades. Computers were first developed in the early 1960s through experiments at the Massachusetts Institute of Technology (MIT) and companies such as The Rand Corporation and IBM. By the mid-1960s the first "minicomputers," which were small enough to sit on a desktop, were developed, as was the Advanced Research Projects Agency Network (ARPANET). ARPANET incorporated the new communication form's technique of "packet switching," which allowed a data system to use one communications link to communicate with more than one machine by disassembling data into datagrams and then gathering these as packets. This major shift in computer communication capabilities revolutionized personal commuting (Computer History Museum, 2010).

The first sites that allowed computer users to interact were primitive bulletin board sites introduced in the late 1970s. Originally these were primarily hosted on personal computers, and users had to dial in through the host computer's modem. Only one person at a time could gain access to the bulletin board (Chapman, 2010). Commercial services that allowed home users to access the Internet for prices that were not prohibitive were introduced in the 1980s, but these services were not available in all areas of the country. By the mid-1990s, however, other online services were available, and home access to the Internet was becoming much more common (Bourne & Bellardo Hahn, 2003). For example, LISTSERV was actually an individual company started in 1985 and was registered as a trademark in 1996. Now offered by various commercial providers, the use of Listservs (as well as forums) has flourished in the 21st century (L-Soft, 2010).

Common Virtual Work Tools

The forms of online and wireless communication and the virtual work tools available to us are in a constant state of evolution. In fact, by the time this chapter is published, it will likely be out of date! However, some of what we are using today is likely to endure, even if improvements and efficiencies are made. With that in mind, the most common types of virtual communication work tools are discussed next.

LISTSERVS

As noted above, LISTSERV® is a proprietary product that has been replicated by programs developed by other software development vendors. These programs allow a person or organization to create, manage, and control electronic mailing lists of recipients who wish to communicate more easily with multiple people at the same time. Whether public and operated through a social media site or private and operated by an individual or an organization, someone typically sets rules about who may join the list (Indiana University Information Technology Services, 2008).

Listserv mailing lists allow people to share and obtain information from multiple sources with minimum effort. All users need to do is write a single e-mail to communicate at low cost with professionals all over the world or make new contacts with persons sharing similar interests they may not otherwise have encountered. Listservs often allow participants to customize how they receive information (e.g., do you want messages automatically delivered to your e-mail in-box, or do you wish to go to a corresponding bulletin board site to read messages?) to make communication more convenient.

VIRTUAL LIVE MEETINGS

Virtual live meetings are conducted using Web conferencing software or Web sites that allow you to meet with others and collaborate in real time over long distances using the Internet. Using this format you can deliver a presentation, collaborate and edit documents, or hold a typical business meeting while physically being in different locations. Such meetings typically require a paid subscription to a service and often combine the use of a personal computer with a traditional conference call. Participants call a toll-free number and log in to a Web site using a link provided to them. The moderator of the conference runs the meeting much as if it were being held in person.

While convenient and highly effective if you are experienced in their use, such Web conferencing meetings can be difficult to manage when the number of participants involved is large, as verbal interchange and discussion become much more complicated to manage. As with any meeting conducted on the telephone, while you can hear participants and benefit from cues such as tone of voice, you cannot see the other participants, so you have limited access to elements of paralanguage, which can increase the risk of misunderstandings.

SOCIAL MEDIA SITES

Social media sites such as Facebook or OT Connections combine multiple virtual communication formats such as bulletin boards or forums for threaded discussions, blogs, and groups for persons sharing common interests, as well as the ability to post pictures and status posting for participants to let others know what they are doing. A major advantage of these sites is that they are free and easily accessible through the Internet. The sites typically allow users to set privacy parameters or offer various parts of the site with differing levels of access. For example, OT Connections has open forums in which both AOTA members and nonmembers can participate, and closed forums accessible only to AOTA members. Because OT Connections is operated by AOTA, it is often used to conduct various types of asynchronous meetings. An asynchronous meeting involves messages that are shared at various times, and posters are not at their computers viewing the same information at the same time.

Pitfalls and Cautions

There are cautions to be heeded when participating in virtual meetings or on social media sites. Virtual written communication is often informal, and this increases the likelihood that misunderstandings may occur. You can easily and unintentionally insult others and must remain aware that you lose control of information once you post it; it becomes permanent and impossible to retract or control who sees it. These sites can blur the lines of personal and professional communication, so you should use them with caution.

Do not fall into the trap of thinking that participating in a virtual meeting is the same as having face-to-face dialogue. When you are speaking with someone face to face you can quickly get feedback on how your message is being received. If you realize that your word choice, tone of voice, or intonation is resulting in an unexpected response or that the impact of your communication is different from what was intended, you can respond and make a correction. However, this is not so easily done online. You may not be able to reach everyone who has read your words to attempt to make a correction. During the time that passes between when readers read your message and when they read your correction, you may have made an indelible impression. You must remember that "what goes on the Net, stays on the Net." There may be a permanent record of your word choice that you may regret later.

> **Virtual written communication is often informal, and this increases the likelihood that misunderstandings may occur. You can easily and unintentionally insult others and must remain aware that you lose control of information once you post it; it becomes permanent and impossible to retract or control who sees it.**

Just as people may type and send an e-mail containing an angry message they would never say in person, sometimes participants in virtual meetings exhibit behavior that they might not if they were in a room and able to see the other participants. It takes an extra level of awareness to realize that when you are staring at an inanimate computer screen and typing on a keyboard, you are still speaking to another human being. Strategies for addressing behavior such as this are presented later in this chapter.

Developing a Virtual Presence: Skills and Strategies

Whether you are running a synchronous 1-hour virtual meeting or an asynchronous meeting that spans days or weeks, a first consideration is to develop an online presence or persona. The concept of a persona technically applies to the idea of playing a character in a play or movie, and while this might not seem genuine or real at first, you will find it much more difficult to always just be yourself in the virtual world. In many instances you may be running meetings with participants who have never met you face to face.

Interpersonal communication styles such as sarcasm in humor that might be effective when a listener can see you and tell from your grin that you are joking can be extremely problematic when interacting over the Internet.

As a leader or as a participant it is important to understand that there are stated, or explicit, rules and unstated (tacit), or implicit, rules to online communication. Implicit rules are often related to the culture of the group or organization in which the meeting is occurring. Group cultures include the values and beliefs that drive shared understanding about rites, rituals, and behaviors, and because these beliefs are frequently unwritten, it can be easy to violate them. One dramatic example of the use of explicit rules are groups that use *Robert's Rules of Order* (Robert, Evans, Honemann, & Ralch, 2000). *Robert's Rules* outline parliamentary procedure for running a meeting and provide in-depth and specific suggestions for such processes as how business is brought before a group, what constitutes a meeting, how decisions are made, and when a group can revisit prior decisions. Due to their extreme complexity, these rules must be used by a meeting leader who has invested time in studying and learning them.

Before running your first virtual meeting, think about who will be attending. Do you know all of the participants and do you have an established relationship, or will this be your first opportunity to make an impression? Think about your first posts and interactions as an opportunity to create your own personal *brand image*. The notion of a brand is that psychological associations such as feelings, beliefs, and attitudes can become associated with the focus of the brand—the product, organization, or, in this case, the person. So consider carefully—what psychological reaction do you want members of a virtual meeting or community to have when they see an e-mail or post from you?

Getting a virtual meeting off to a good start can be a lot like starting a meeting when the members are in the same room. Here are a few suggestions for running effective face-to-face meetings that can also be used in virtual meetings:

- Distribute an agenda in advance of the start of the meeting with discussion items listed and include a time frame for each item.
- Clearly state the start and end times of the meeting and do not deviate from these times without the agreement of group members.
- Establish ground rules to guide meeting behavior, such as being logged on and "in" the meeting before the stated start time and having all phones on "mute" so that the meeting is not disturbed by background noise.

- Decide how members will indicate that they wish to ask a question or comment. Are you using a system (in synchronous meetings) that allows someone to virtually "raise their hand"?
- Decide how you will decide. How will decisions be made? Do you have time to work for consensus, or will you allow decision making by voting? If you will be voting, will members vote publicly?
- Consider starting the meeting with an icebreaker if members are new to one another. This can vary from simple introductions to sharing more in-depth information about each person's background and experience.

Once a meeting is established and an agenda and ground rules have been set, it is time to consider online behaviors in running the meeting.

Virtual Meeting Rules and How to Handle Renegades

Like any meeting, it is helpful to establish rules that guide behavior for virtual meetings. These rules are in addition to the ground rules previously suggested and are related to more specific behaviors. For example, a general ground rule might be that you vote only on less important issues and attempt to reach consensus for critical decisions. However, when you do vote it will be important to have rules on how this is done. For example, how many hours will participants have to vote? Will you consider accepting votes submitted after the deadline or after voting is closed? Issues like this are more important when running asynchronous meetings than when you can stop and check with all participants for approval during a synchronous meeting.

For example, the Representative Assembly (RA), which is the policy-making body for AOTA, uses *Robert's Rules* when official meetings are conducted, whether face to face or online. The level of importance of the business conducted by the RA has motivated AOTA on occasion to hire a trained and certified parliamentarian to consult with the leader of the group (the Speaker) and to be present at all official meetings of the RA. Other groups, ranging from occupational therapy departments to condominium association boards of directors, may use a less-formal approach but often do rely on such elements of *Robert's Rules* as requiring a "second" on a motion before agreeing to discuss it. Whether or not a meeting leader is prepared to fully implement *Robert's Rules*, what is most important is having a preestablished set of rules that are understood by all participants and consistently applied.

So what happens when meeting participants break a rule? First, be clear that violations of the rules *will* happen, whether intentionally or unintentionally. If your preestablished rules address violations, you have a place to start. When using *Robert's Rules,* the meeting leader might declare the person violating a rule to be "out of order" and redirect the group to accepted behavior and the business at hand. In less-formal situations the leader might gently call attention to the violation of the rule and suggest that the participants refocus.

If you have participated in virtual meetings you may be thinking, "Hold on. That is easy in a synchronous meeting when the leader can get everyone's attention at once. What do you do when someone breaks a rule in an asynchronous meeting?" That question would highlight a difficulty of running meetings that are longer than an hour or two when you can communicate the same information to everyone at the same time. When using an asynchronous format such as OT Connections and running a meeting over days, or in the case of the RA, weeks, maintaining order and addressing a violation of procedures produce a particular type of challenge to the leader. What are the primary strategies in this case?

Unfortunately the most straightforward answer is time, attention, and commitment. Using virtual meeting formats such as Live Meeting or OT Connections can save an organization considerable resources such as travel expenses and travel time. However, that payoff may be offset by the additional time and resources incurred by those running and supporting the meeting. For example, while State Representatives may spend 30 to 60 minutes a day checking in on an online RA meeting, the Speaker and the AOTA staff person who supports the meeting may have to spend hours checking in for new posts each day that the meeting runs. An unexpected implication of this meeting format is that while overall resources may be saved, it may place unintentional limits on who may be willing to volunteer for leadership roles.

It may sound like running an extended virtual meeting is almost an impossible task, and it certainly is complicated. However, there are strategies that can help. Among many, a few of the most useful include the following:

1. Distribute formal "Rules of the Day" to guide meeting behavior in addition to the general ground rules (see Figure 16.1 for a sample Rules of the Day for a prolonged meeting).
2. If you are the leader of a virtual meeting, plan ahead and block out specific times in your schedule to go online.

3. Identify formal coleaders or informal "watchers" who agree to check the posts in the meeting frequently and alert you by e-mail of minor problems or by phone or text message if your immediate attention is required.

4. Establish rules and shared expectations about "offline" communication outside of the meeting. Is it okay for members to communicate, share information, or debate out of the confines of the virtual meeting (i.e., behind the scenes)? Is it understood that it is acceptable for you as the meeting leader to contact meeting participants individually through e-mail, phone, or text message? Doing this allows you to gently redirect minor rule violations.

5. Consider building a break or days off into the meeting schedule to allow you and coleaders to regroup or problem-solve.

6. Build extra days into the meeting schedule to allow you to extend the meeting if necessary. Use these extra days only if it is absolutely critical.

7. Expect your level of stress to increase, and be sure you have support so that you can keep your cool.

When you believe that inappropriate behavior or rule-breaking might be unintentional or that a participant's emotions may have temporarily overridden common sense, consider sending a gentle message either publicly or privately. If the participant is unaware, he or she may immediately self-correct and change the behavior and even apologize to the group.

Sometimes, however, rule-breaking or other such behavior is intentional, and this calls for more assertive action on the part of the group leader. You might wonder why a group member would intentionally break a rule. Even in a professional working group, renegades who may be well intentioned might be convinced that they must skirt the established rules to ensure that information is brought before the group, that a decision is influenced, or that the group change course. Some very experienced members who are familiar with *Robert's Rules* or other forms of parliamentary procedure or who are very comfortable with virtual meetings may still become

> **When you believe that inappropriate behavior or rule-breaking might be unintentional or that a participant's emotions may have temporarily overridden common sense, consider sending a gentle message either publicly or privately.**

AOTA

Rules of the Online Meeting of the Representative Assembly (RA)
Fall Meeting with Discussion Items

1. The Speaker shall call for the Online Meeting and shall state the dates and times the meeting will be called to order and adjourned.

2. Members shall sign in for a roll call ("RA Member Roll Call") with their name, position, and election area within the first 24 hours of the Online Meeting. Members include: Representatives, Alternate Representatives, RA Officials, AOTA Committee/Commission/Council Chairs and Chair-Elects, OTs in Foreign Countries (OTFC) Representative, Affiliated State Association Presidents (ASAP) Representative, Assembly of Student Delegates (ASD) Representative, Occupational Therapy Assistant (OTA) Representative and OTA Alternate Representative to the Assembly, RA Committee Chairs, Consumer Member, AOTA Officers and Officers-Elect, and the AOTA Executive Director.

3. Members properly credentialed have speaking privileges. Only Representatives, AOTA Committee/Commission/Council Chairs, RA Officials, OTFC Representative, ASAP Representative, ASD Representative, OTA Representative, Consumer Member, and AOTA Officers may vote.

4. Resource persons including AOTA staff may be asked to respond to requests for information and/or clarification upon invitation of the Speaker.

5. The Recorder shall report a quorum. When a quorum is established, the Speaker shall call the meeting to order. Another quorum does not need to be established during the Online Meeting. If RA members join the meeting after the quorum is established, they shall notify the Credential Review and Accountability Committee (CRAC) Chair through the "RA Member Roll Call." The CRAC Chair shall keep a record of the attendance of voting and nonvoting members.

6. The Agenda Chair shall present the Consent Agenda and/or Main Agenda for consideration during the Online Meeting.

7. As motions are made, time stamp indicated on the Web Board in EST allows them to be handled in order.

8. The first person addressing the motion constitutes a second.

9. Members may post only two times on a motion unless responding to requests for information or requests for clarification and have been recognized by the Speaker.

FIGURE 16.1. Sample Rules of the Day for an online meeting.

10. When a member makes an amendment, it must be clearly identified and postings should be made to the amendment. Discussion on the main motion must stop until the amendment is resolved. Tracking of amendments may be assigned to any of the RA Officials by the Speaker.

11. The first person addressing an amendment constitutes a second. If there is no second within 24 hours of the amendment, the amendment is automatically defeated and discussion returns to the main motion.

12. If debate on a motion or an amendment cannot be completed within the scheduled time for the meeting, a member of the Assembly or the Speaker may move to postpone the discussion until a future meeting of the Assembly.

13. No more than two additional motions will be considered to an original motion before it is automatically referred to a future meeting of the Assembly.

14. A member may call a point of order or appeal from the decision of the Speaker. The appeal shall be sent to an Appeals Committee which shall include the Recorder and two seated voting RA members.

15. Votes shall be taken by the Recorder using roll call on the meeting site. The minutes shall reflect only the final tallies.

16. Voting Procedures:

    a. Voting on the Rules of the Day for the Online Meeting shall be completed within the time indicated on the agenda for this item of business. The results of the vote shall be reported to the Speaker by the Recorder and announced to the Assembly, at which time the Rules shall be in effect.

    b. Motions on the Main Agenda shall be considered in the order designated and within the time set by the Agenda Chair. The Speaker shall call the vote on amendments within the period of debate scheduled for that main motion.

    c. Voting on motions must be done by RA members within 24 hours of the Speaker's closing debate specific to each motion. Votes submitted after the 24 hours will not be accepted. Member voting is to be done on each motion in their individual segments of the meeting site.

    d. When voting, a majority means "more than half" of the votes cast. In the case of a required two-thirds vote, it will be by two-thirds of the votes cast.

17. The Recorder and CRAC Chair shall serve as tellers and shall submit all vote tallies to the Speaker no later than 96 hours after the close of the Online Meeting. The Speaker shall report the results to the Assembly and the Recorder shall report the results to the members of AOTA in the minutes.

FIGURE 16.1. Sample Rules of the Day for an online meeting. (*Cont.*)

renegades. A few strategies for responding to a renegade and intentional or unintentional rule-breaking include the following:

1. Be direct, immediate, and public in your response. Let the entire group know that you are aware that a rule has been broken.
2. Quickly assess the tone you intend to convey in your response. If the violation is minor, humor might be appropriate and may result in the group quickly returning to business as usual. If the violation is more serious, individual contact by e-mail or phone might be appropriate.
3. If you have any question about whether a rule is being broken, consult with a coleader or trusted member of the group to validate or invalidate your concern.
4. Rely on formally identified coleaders. If another member of the group identifies and corrects behavior, you may not be put in the position of always being the "bad guy" or "sheriff."
5. If a person's behavior becomes repetitive and problematic, do not ignore it. Use formal channels to make the individual aware that you and others see the behavior as a problem, explicitly state what behavior is expected in the future, and document this interaction.

Managing Agendas

Earlier the suggestion was made that one strategy for running an effective virtual meeting is to distribute an agenda in advance. Agendas are common, and almost anyone who has participated in formal meetings will be familiar with them. However, when running a virtual meeting, particularly an asynchronous meeting that extends over days or weeks, there are new considerations. For example, do you have only one discussion occurring at a time, or do you schedule multiple discussion threads that overlap? If you are conducting the meeting formally using parliamentary procedures, how much time do you schedule for discussion and for voting, and how will you manage amendments or other points of order that may come up? Will you make use of a consent agenda, in which multiple items are grouped together and given an "up or down" vote as a block (members are typically given a chance to remove items from a consent agenda to place them on the main agenda for discussion)? Answering these questions will likely be influenced by the number of participants and their familiarity with your group process, with each other and the work at hand, and the time commitment expected from members.

For example, AOTA has several groups that run virtual meetings each year. Some of these groups handle multiple items of business within a single meeting, with each item requiring a period of discussion and debate, some items that allow for amendments to motions to be made, and time for a vote. Each activity often extends over a 48-hour period, so from start to finish a single item of business may take 4 or 5 days to complete. If a group has multiple business items, the meeting can take a long time. To avoid this, the meeting agendas typically call for the introduction of several items for discussion. As these discussions take shape and move toward a period of voting, new items are introduced in a staggered manner. An example of an agenda for a multiday meeting of AOTA's RA is included in Figure 16.2.

PREPARING GROUP MEMBERS TO EFFECTIVELY HANDLE VIRTUAL MEETING AGENDAS AND BUSINESS

Preparing members for participation in a virtual meeting or for conducting ongoing business online can be a formidable task. However, the more prepared and the better informed the participants are, the more likely they will be able to actively contribute to your group. Helping to prepare group members for virtual work goes beyond setting ground rules and shared expectations and creating an agenda. It is also important to technically prepare members. You must make sure that participants have the necessary hardware and software and access to be online at the right times. Some participants may need technical assistance to download and use the software needed for some online meeting formats, and reliable Internet access may be an issue for some participants.

While using platforms like OT Connections may come naturally and seem intuitive for participants already familiar with other social media sites, those new to such formats may struggle with finding the meeting and posting, or they may be confused when multiple discussions are occurring at the same time. Here are a few strategies for helping to prepare your participants for a virtual meeting:

1. Send directions for joining the meeting several days in advance, and perhaps send them multiple times to ensure all participants receive the information. If the meeting makes use of a Web conferencing system that

2009 Fall Online Representative Assembly

Requests to remove an item from the Consent Agenda must be made by **October 28 (9 a.m. EST)**. SHADED indicates timeline for Online Meeting if no items are removed from the Consent Agenda. Information in ( ) indicates probable time frame if items are removed from the Consent Agenda.

DATE	DISCUSSION	VOTING
November 2 Start Time: **9:00 a.m. EST** Monday	**OPENING DAY** • (Agenda Item #1 – only if an item is removed from the Consent Agenda)	• **Consent Agenda (Opens 9 a.m. EST)**
November 3 Tuesday	• (Agenda Item #1)	• **Consent Agenda**
November 4 Wednesday	**CLOSING DAY** • (Agenda Item #2 – only if an item is removed from the Consent Agenda)	• **Consent Agenda (Closes 9 a.m. EST)** • (Agenda Item #1 – only if an item is removed from the Consent Agenda)
November 5 Thursday	• (Agenda Item #2)	• (Agenda Item #1)
November 6 Friday		• (Agenda Item #2 – only if an item is removed from the Consent Agenda)
November 7 Saturday		• (Agenda Item #2)
November 8 Sunday	• (Closing Day)	
November 9 Monday	Please keep these days open in case business is extended by an amendment	
November 10 Tuesday		
November 11 Wednesday		
November 12 Thursday		
November 13 Friday		

FIGURE 16.2. Sample AOTA Representative Assembly online meeting agenda and timeline.

requires downloading software, inform participants that all software needs to be downloaded and working properly ahead of the meeting.

2. Offer a training session that demonstrates the Web conferencing program or social media site to be used. Send screenshots if possible to make directions clearer.

3. Establish a practice site. If you will be running multiple discussion threads, set up at least two mock discussions and have participants practice posting.

4. Ask that all participants be "at" the meeting (i.e., sign on and call in) 15 minutes before your first meeting.

5. For large groups include several volunteers who will be willing to work one to one with participants who have trouble. The volunteers can call participants who are struggling and walk them through any problematic procedure.

Even with the best training and participation you should expect problems, especially with large groups. For example, participants who ignore requests to do a trial run of joining a meeting and then attempt to sign on from a work site the day of the meeting may learn that they do not have the administrative rights to download the necessary software for Web conferencing. In addition, Web conferencing software and Web sites are sometimes updated, and new software may need to be downloaded or a site may look different than when last visited! So, train your participants, but expect that you might have problems.

MANAGING BUSINESS HOUR BY HOUR OR DAY BY DAY

There are also strategies you can use to help things go smoothly when you are ready to prepare your first agenda. Most important, think "big picture" first! What is the purpose of the meeting? Are the participants all familiar with this purpose and on the same page, or would they benefit from some orientation? What must be achieved by the end of the meeting? If you do not achieve your desired outcomes will you have another opportunity? What pace should you set for business? These are just a few of the big-picture questions that should guide the planning of your agenda.

As noted, an agenda should be planned and distributed in advance. For a short meeting that may last only an hour or so you should carefully consider how much business you will be able to achieve. Moreover, consider your group's behavior. How many of your participants are truly likely to be signed in and ready to go at the designated time? Waiting and starting late to accommodate tardy participants may only reinforce this behavior, whereas starting on time even if you are missing a few participants rewards those who are on time and helps establish the shared expectation of being on time. If your meeting will extend over a period of days or weeks, consider starting the meeting with something procedural or a less important item of business to work out the kinks and allow all participants to become oriented to the meeting forum.

For these longer meetings, participants may find it useful if you help to orient them as business evolves by doing daily announcements that remind them of critical steps to be taken each day, such as "Discussion on Agenda Item 4 begins today!" or "Don't forget that voting on the Motion to Create a New Web site ends today!" As suggested earlier, allowing some time for breaks to regroup and for some additional time that you will use only if you need it, and planning for unfinished business, are important strategies for effectively managing an agenda.

CONCLUDING BUSINESS: SET THE TONE FOR THE FUTURE

Some meetings go better than others, and even the most experienced leader can have a meeting during which it seems that almost everything goes wrong. Regardless of how well or poorly a meeting goes or if it is your first or 50th virtual meeting, you should plan to end it formally. This helps to leave the participants with a sense of satisfaction and to be better prepared for the next meeting and the work ahead.

Concluding, or "wrapping up," a virtual meeting is much like ending a face-to-face meeting, and there are several commonsense steps that you should take. First, confirm that everyone is in agreement that the planned business has been concluded. This may seem like a simple step, but in a complicated meeting (face-to-face or virtual), it is easy to indicate that you will come back to a suggestion or question but then lose track. One helpful strategy is to keep a public posting, or "parking lot," of any questions or business that are off the topic currently being discussed and to have the group view this list and decide how to proceed before adjourning.

Second, give participants an opportunity to identify business that they would like to have added to the next meeting. Making this list public during the meeting may also be a cue to help participants stay on topic. Finally, consider the "thank you" or other messages you may want to share before adjourning. Thank those who made special contributions and any first-timers for attending, and acknowledge any participant who may be leaving the group. Again, think about what you would do if you had worked for several days with participants in a face-to-face meeting, and consider how to translate these actions to the virtual world.

> **Thank those who made special contributions and any first-timers for attending, and acknowledge any participant who may be leaving the group. Again, think about what you would do if you had worked for several days with participants in a face-to-face meeting, and consider how to translate these actions to the virtual world.**

A final example of this behavior is to conduct some type of formal assessment of the meeting, including what worked well and what should be changed. Did the participants have difficulty with the technology? Did new members receive an appropriate orientation? Were the pace and the length of the meeting appropriate, or was it too slow, too fast, too short, or too long? As with any meeting evaluation, you may have to consider this feedback in the context of the changes you have control over. For instance, if a participant criticizes the basic approach of having a virtual meeting, is there anything you can do to address this? You may not be able to change the meeting to a face-to-face meeting, but you can go back to this participant to see what would improve his or her experience.

If you have formal or informal coleaders of the meeting or a support person who aids you with the logistics of the meeting, it is highly valuable to spend time processing how things went as soon as the meeting is concluded. Keep a brief daily journal or notes about things that worked or about what to do differently the next time. If you do daily announcements, keep an electronic copy so that you don't have to reinvent these from scratch for the next meeting. In addition, if you will be turning over responsibility for running the meeting to someone else in the future, the new leader will certainly benefit from and appreciate your hard work. While it may be hard to focus on this task immediately after a long meeting, it is important to process before you forget the most salient experiences. Doing this small piece of work now will benefit you in the future and make it more likely that your future virtual meetings will become even more effective.

Mastering a New Form of Writing

The advent of the Internet, wireless technologies, and other virtual work environments and tools has forever changed the way that some day-to-day business is conducted. While there are clear advantages in terms of the time and financial resources saved when travel is avoided, there are also new challenges that result, particularly for leaders of virtual meetings. Many of the common strategies and behaviors associated with running effective face-to-face meetings can be migrated to the virtual world. The use of agendas, ground rules, and careful consideration of word choice and clear organization of ideas will help you in the running of a virtual meeting.

New strategies must also be adopted that are specific to a virtual meeting. You may have participants who have never met face to face before, and you also must vary the strategies you use depending on whether participants are experiencing the same communication at the same time in a synchronous meeting or may be reading and posting at different times of the day in an asynchronous meeting. Combining longstanding approaches to running effective meetings with evolving strategies for operating in the virtual world can be challenging, but as virtual meetings become more commonplace, there are more and more resources available to guide you. Take advantage of these resources, and network with others in your professional community to help you learn the skills and strategies you'll need for designing a productive meeting as well as avoiding common pitfalls.

REFERENCES

Bourne, C. P., & Bellardo Hahn, T. (2003). *A history of online information services, 1963–1976*. Cambridge, MA: MIT Press.

Chapman, C. (2010). *The history and evolution of social media*. Retrieved from http://www.webdesignerdepot.com/2009/10/the-history-and-evolution-of-social-media

Computer History Museum. (2010). *A history of the Internet: 1962–1992*. Retrieved from http://www.computerhistory.org/internet_history/index.html

Gates, B. (n.d.). Retrieved from http://sourcesofinsight.com/lessons-learned-from-bill-gates

Indiana University Information Technology Services. (2008). *What is a LISTSERV mailing list?* Retrieved from http://kb.iu.edu/data/afah.html

L-Soft. (2010). *History of LISTSERV*. Retrieved from http://www.lsoft.com/corporate/history_listserv.asp

Robert, H. M., Evans, W. J., Honemann, D. H., & Ralch, T. J. (2000). *Robert's rules of order: Newly revised* (10th ed.). Cambridge, MA: Da Capo Press.

Netiquette: Communicating Effectively on the Internet

FRAN BABISS, PhD, OTR/L

The Internet could be a very positive step towards education, organisation and participation in a meaningful society.

—Noam Chomsky (2002)

The Internet has changed our world, and it will continue to do so. E-mails, text messages, and tweets have nearly replaced stamped letters. Few think twice about using computers and smartphones to communicate and obtain information. To be effective in this new world, occupational therapy practitioners need to understand how to successfully and safely communicate using these new technologies.

What is netiquette? *Netiquette,* a combination of the words *network* and *etiquette,* refers to the rules for proper behavior on the Internet (Wikipedia, 2011a). The term came into being in the mid-1990s as the Internet began to grow and become accessible to more than just a few engineering and defense experts. Computers are now an indispensable and legitimate communication tool for occupational therapy practitioners, and learning the rules for communicating by means of this new domain is essential for those who wish to remain professionally viable.

> If you already communicate politely and effectively over the phone, on paper, at meetings, and in other contexts, much of what you already do is appropriate in the digital environment.

There's another reason occupational therapy practitioners need to be familiar with the customs of the new technology. Attitudes toward digital communication may contribute to a collision of generations (Lancaster & Stillman, 2002) as individuals strive to adapt to a rapidly changing world. For example, a fieldwork student texts a question to her supervisor, who doesn't know how to text back. A Boomer-aged occupational therapist invites a Millennial intern to be her friend on Facebook, but the intern sees this as an intrusion into his private life. A young occupational therapist thanks a retiring supervisor in an e-mail, unaware that the supervisor expected a handwritten note. Such differences in perspective are being negotiated in occupational therapy settings every day.

If you already communicate politely and effectively over the phone, on paper, at meetings, and in other contexts, much of what you already do is appropriate in the digital environment. This chapter discusses what you also need to know to be professional and follow the rules of netiquette when communicating in writing online. It covers what netiquette is, the contexts in which it is used, and ways to maintain safety in a computer world.

A chapter like this may be unnecessary in the future, but online communication is still relatively new, and rules of etiquette develop over time. Occupational therapy practitioners who grew up in the era preceding the ubiquity of computers will learn how to use them to communicate more effectively. For those who hail from more recent generations, this chapter provides a refresher on the rules of etiquette in the digital world.

Brief History of Netiquette

After the World Wide Web came into widespread use around 1993, the number of people using it grew quickly. America Online was one of the first of many companies to make it easy to connect to the Internet, allowing people with similar interests all over the world instant access to one another. In chat rooms, for example, people participated in real-time discussions, formed relationships, and interacted in a way that clearly required rules for proper decorum. The early days of the Internet have been compared to the Wild West, where in the popular imagination anything was allowed, and people could act freely without fear of reprisal (Morriss, 1998).

The impact of negative behavior in an ungoverned environment led to the creation of rules for network etiquette. In October 1995, Sally Hambridge of Intel Corporation released a memorandum on the subject of netiquette that is considered to be the first document of its kind.

By the late 1990s, the Internet had evolved to feature many new opportunities for interoperability, interaction, and user-centered design; the term *Web 2.0* was coined to describe this more sophisticated environment (Wikipedia, 2011b). Web 2.0 gave rise to the social media, and opportunities to express oneself, in good ways and bad, have proliferated. As new platforms for communication have been developed, new rules have been born.

Netiquette Contexts

The suggestions in this section represent a synthesis from respected online sources such as the Yale University Library (2007) and Shea's (1997) netiquette Web site, along with my own experiences as an occupational therapist and user of the Internet.

E-MAIL

The first network e-mail was sent in 1971 by Ray Tomlinson (n.d.), an American defense employee, launching a new era in business and personal communication. In many ways, writing an e-mail message is similar to writing a letter. A salutation begins the message, it's followed by the body of the message and a closing such as "Sincerely," and the sender's name and contact information complete the message. A few rules have evolved to help e-mail writers more effectively convey their message:

- *Think before you hit "send."* Daniel Goleman, author of *Emotional Intelligence* (1997), noted in a *New York Times* essay (2007) that the lack of nonverbal clues normally available in face-to-face communication can easily lead your readers to misconstrue the tone or even the content of your message. Reread your message before you send it, listening for how your audience will hear it and tweaking to be sure readers will understand what you want to convey.

- *Use the customary rules of grammar and mechanics, and always proofread before sending.* You are representing your personal and professional identity in an e-mail, and spelling and grammar count. Writing in all lowercase letters or with errors in punctuation will not reflect well on you. Likewise, the use of all capital letters may be interpreted as the equivalent of shouting. Take a moment to carefully reread each e-mail before you send it, considering how you would feel if it were to resurface 5 years from now. E-mail, especially if connected with a large organization, may be archived permanently.

- *Use the "Reply to All" feature sparingly.* Many e-mails sent to groups of people require a response only to the sender. Replying to all is appropriate if all recipients need to know how the others respond, but unnecessary use makes for a long thread of responses and clutters in-boxes with irrelevant e-mails.

- *Make the subject line of your e-mail meaningful.* I received an e-mail from an occupational therapy intern a few years ago with the subject "Can you help?" I had no way to know what the e-mail was about, beyond a plea for help. A brief but detailed subject line helps the recipient to find the e-mail later.

- *Do not forward joke or chain e-mails at work.* There are so many funny and heartwarming e-mails that circulate on the Internet, and nearly all of us receive them from time to time. If you just have to share them, send them from your personal e-mail account to the recipient's personal account. Work is not the place for these. My hospital's computer department asks us to resist forwarding these types of e-mails, as it wastes storage space. It is important to realize as well that people with malicious intent may gather e-mail addresses using forwarded messages.

- *To orient readers, quote the parts of the message you are responding to.* I generally use copy and paste when referencing the parts of another person's e-mail I want to respond to. Some e-mail programs have ways to automate this procedure.

- *It is often better to handle complicated negotiations and topics face to face or over the telephone.* If you and your correspondent e-mail back and forth several times, it might be time to communicate by another means. E-mail threads that become very long can be complicated to follow. In most e-mail programs, the older material is at the bottom of the inter-change, which can confuse the reader.

- *Do not forward a personal e-mail without the author's permission.* What a person has written to you may be intended for you only. I once received an e-mail complaint from a peer and without thinking forwarded it to the person it concerned, thinking I was expediting the process of getting the information sent to the person in question. This was a breach of confidentiality, and it took several months, an apology, and a meeting with the three people involved to straighten it out. What a person sends to you is to be considered confidential and is for your eyes only unless you have permission to forward it.

- *Use the "Blind Carbon Copy" (Bcc:) feature to protect others' e-mail addresses.* I paste the e-mail addresses into the "Bcc:" (rather than the "To:") line to protect the identity and privacy of the people to whom I am sending a group e-mail. Most mail services have an option to send e-mail this way.

- *Emoticons are not professional but can be used in special instances.* Emoticons are pictorial representations of emotion that are formed us-ing keyboard symbols—for example, :-) for a smiley face—to denote mood and intent. Your writing should communicate your intent using words alone. With coworkers with whom I have a close relationship, I use emoticons, but I think before I use them: Is this a person with whom I have an emotional connection? If I were responding to a query from a publisher, as I did when I agreed to write this chapter, emoticons would have been inappropriately informal.

DISCUSSION GROUPS

The first large-scale human interactions on the Internet after network e-mail came with the advent of discussion groups. A discussion group is generally limited to a specific topic, and members of the group can post (i.e., type and send) their own contributions on the topic and respond to other posts. There are discussion groups on any subject you can think of.

To read the postings in a newsgroup an individual had to have special newsreader software. This made the information inaccessible to most peo-ple, for whom this process was too cumbersome and technical. In the late 1990s this writer belonged to newsgroups on graphic typography—what are often called *fonts*. An individual would write a question or a comment and send it to an address that communicated with the Usenet, and their letter or

> Thinking before you hit "send," using the customary rules of grammar and mechanics, proofreading your posts, and quoting the part of a post you are responding to will ensure that you are a welcome member of the discussion.

post would appear on the Internet on a location where the newsgroup had a page. Members of the group can go to that page to look at the posts from their peers, and respond to or comment on the posts that were grouped there.

As a way of getting a message or request out to many people, discussion groups are a great tool. Usenet newsgroups, bulletin boards, and listservs have been popular ways of sharing information among groups of people, but for the most part, forums have evolved as the most common type of discussion group.

A forum is a great resource for group problem-solving and online discussion of specific topics. Forums are usually maintained in one place and may have a human moderator whose task is to ensure the politeness of the group, the relevance of the posts, and the quality of the material. The American Occupational Therapy Association (AOTA) has forums on its OT Connections Web site (http://otconnections.aota.org/) for the Special Interest Sections and on many topics of interest to the occupational therapy community. Many of the OT Connections forums are open to anyone, regardless of membership in AOTA. These forums offer a wealth of information and interaction on many facets of the profession.

As in e-mails, thinking before you hit "send," using the customary rules of grammar and mechanics, proofreading your posts, and quoting the part of a post you are responding to will ensure that you are a welcome member of the discussion. In addition, the following rules will help you use forums effectively (Thompson, 2007):

- *Read the FAQs.* Nearly all forums list frequently asked questions that will answer many of the questions you have. The list of FAQs provides an introduction to participation in the forum and can help you avoid gaffes. In addition, FAQs have information on whom to contact for help should you need it. On the OT Connections home page (i.e., the first page you see) are links to videos that show you how to create an account (i.e., register) for the forums; you cannot write a forum post without an account. Membership in AOTA automatically allows you to log into (enter) OT Connections using your AOTA name and password, but non-members can also create an account and participate in the forums.

- *Review the questions in the forum before you ask your question, and read entire posts.* Many forums have expert moderators who monitor the questions asked; for example, Tina Champagne, OTD, used to monitor and answer questions on the forum of the Mental Health Special Interest Section. Imagine how much work she would have if she had to repeatedly answer questions about where mental health jobs can be found! First review what has already been posted to see if your question has been answered, and take the time to read the entire post—not just scan it—to ensure that if the answer to your question is there, you'll find it. Most forums allow searches for terms related to a query. Often, the search can be done using key words, the name of the author of the posts, or the date of the post.

- *Post under the appropriate category.* The OT Connections forum categories are specific. Of course, you may ask your question in two places—for example, in the Administration and Management forum and in the Gerontology forum—if your question spans both of those areas.

- *Avoid netspeak.* All languages have their slang, and Internet slang, or *netspeak,* is a special form of argot; lol (laughing out loud), OMG (oh my God), and other forms of shorthand are everywhere on the Internet. Netspeak is most appropriate in communications where brevity is an asset, such as in instant messaging, some social network media, and a virtual world (discussed later in this chapter). In forum postings, however, netspeak is informal and unprofessional and should be avoided.

- *Do not double post.* It is easy to hit "send" twice; if you do so, your message will be posted twice, annoying fellow group members.

The Wild West ethos of the Internet is alive and well in discussion groups. Occasionally you may come into contact with negative people and behaviors in a forum. The following are suggestions for identifying and avoiding them:

- *Trolls.* A troll is a person who deliberately looks to create conflict and provoke arguments. Trolls are excited by the belief that they have the power to upset forum members. The term *troll,* besides referring to the loutish mythological creature, relates to fishing, as in trolling for suckers—people who will rise to the bait by posting an emotional response. For example, a member posts a question to an OT Connections forum asking for help defending the use of bedside occupational therapy in a nursing home about to cut this service. A troll might post, "Well, occupational therapists have not demonstrated any significant outcomes working bedside, so why should it matter?" This reply would be sure to anger many readers, and those who took the bait would only please the troll, who in so posting has derailed the direction of the original post.

- *Sockpuppets.* The anonymity of the Internet allows people to take on multiple personae through fake accounts. A *sockpuppet* is a type of false identity that forum members could use to make flattering postings about their real identity or denigrating postings about someone with whom they disagree. For example, if someone gives a book a negative review in a forum, the book's author could use a sockpuppet account to post a good review and criticize the negative reviewer. The well-moderated OT Connections forums generally are not plagued with such bothers, but it is best to remain aware that forum members may be hiding their real identities.
- *Flamers.* The *flamer* makes a direct attack on someone in a forum, resulting in a heated debate. When the targeted person reacts, a *flame war* erupts. Well-known flame wars are frequently political, pitting one extreme against another, as in a debate between liberals and conservatives. A flame war might erupt in the Sensory Integration Special Interest Section forum, for example, if a flamer denigrated sensory integration (SI) in favor of applied behavioral analysis and proponents of SI responded equally insultingly.

SOCIAL MEDIA

Every day new forms of social media are being created. Social media, simply put, are technologies people can use in social interaction with others. You may have experience with Flickr, which stores photos; YouTube, which stores videos; podcasts, which are serial audio or audiovisual presentations; and Webinars, which use the Internet to broadcast seminars. Many social media sites cost nothing to join. Because the social media can provide access to huge audiences, people have found ways to use them to gain fame and fortune; for example, those who post a video on YouTube that becomes viral (i.e., ubiquitous) can earn money from advertisers.

The sections that follow discuss the social media that primarily involve written communication—social networking sites, blogs, and messaging—and describe some ways professionals and organizations can use them to reach the public.

Social Networking Sites

Social networking sites are a way to connect with people who are far away, around the corner, or right in your house. Users create their own network and invite others to join. Facebook is the most widely used Web 2.0 tool; it allows users to say what's on their mind and view one another's photos and provides numerous ways to entertain oneself. Like many others, I've found and recommended relationships on Facebook with people I'd lost contact with over the years.

LinkedIn is a similar site with a professional networking focus, and several occupational therapy groups are available on the site, including one for AOTA members. If you seek a professional space to let people know about your occupational therapy practice, and want an inexpensive way to do this, then LinkedIn may meet your needs.

Social networking possibilities expand daily, providing occupational therapists with the tools to reach wider audiences. Sites such as Pinterest or Scoop.it allow anyone to create a pinboard of items that are of interest. "OT mash up" is the pinboard of PhD student Rashid Kashani, displaying visually pleasing and disparate items about the profession such as suggestions of adapted tools for food preparation and information about spinal cord functions (see http://pinterest.com/rkashani/ot-mash-up/). Occupational therapists can use these tools to promote the profession, promote their own services, or to showcase the talents of others.

Twitter enables users to send *tweets*—originally 140-character typed statements—over the Internet to those in their network. Although many tweets are first-person updates about the tweeter's whereabouts or mood or what they're doing or thinking, and therefore of limited relevance, Twitter has also become the place to go for the latest breaking news. I heard about the earthquake in Haiti and the death of Michael Jackson from updates on Twitter. At this writing, Twitter is launching advertising allowing participants to promote themselves and their products. Most of these networks have a follow option, which allows the reader to receive updated information. The more followers a person has, the greater his or her network.

The power afforded by social networks comes with the responsibility of professionals to be polite. As several sports and entertainment celebrities have found, it is always important to think about your potential audience before you post anything to the Internet.

Blogs

Blogs (short for *weblogs*) are Web sites in which a person or group posts commentary about a particular topic. Blogs sometimes include audio and video files, graphics, and links to other Web sites. Visitors to a blog can post their own comments in response to the blog's content.

Anyone can start a blog using free or low-cost tools that are readily available on the Internet. AOTA's Web site has a tab that will take you to a list of blogs created by occupational therapists. A blog can be an opportunity to share your views and beliefs about the profession as well as providing readers with access to comment and dialogue. If you start a blog and want to increase readership, it's incumbent upon you to update often and check comments frequently.

Text Messaging and Instant Messaging

Text messages are brief messages sent by telephone; like e-mail, they are stored and can be retrieved and responded to at the user's convenience. *Instant messaging (IM)*, in contrast, takes place in real time and is more like a written phone conversation; both parties must be on the computer or smartphone at the same time. Shipley and Schwalbe (2007) suggested that IM will surpass e-mail as the main means of communicating in business environments, and many large corporations have Intranet services for employees with IM built in to provide fast access to coworkers in real time.

Suggestions for texting and IM are few but important. Similar to e-mail, these forms of communication make it difficult to express tone and emotion. It is best to use simple language. A few other tips follow:

- *Keep your messages short.* This is not the medium for long dialogues.
- *Ask yourself if the message is appropriate for an instant message or text.* These communications are informal and should not be used for formal situations.
- *Be careful with abbreviations.* Know your audience. Not everyone is familiar with all the shortcuts used in text and instant messages.
- *Do not text confidential material.* There is no way to know who is reading your text message.

VIRTUAL CONTEXTS

Three-dimensional virtual worlds offer opportunities for imaginative and educational applications for occupational therapists (Babiss, 2007). A *virtual world* is a computer-simulated environment in which people can interact and create and use objects. Second Life® is the best known of all the virtual worlds, with a current membership of about half a million *avatars* (i.e., users' bodily representation in Second Life).

One occupational therapist, Dr. Susan Toth-Cohen, PhD, who calls herself Zsuzsa Tomsen in Second Life, is using this platform to educate the public about occupational therapy and to provide her students at Thomas Jefferson University with tools and challenges to get the message out about the value of occupational therapy in contexts such as healthy aging, adaptive equipment, sensory interventions, adaptive playgrounds, and explanations of the science underlying the practice of the profession (see http://maps.secondlife.com/secondlife/Eduisland%202/151/28/22).

Users communicate with others in Second Life by either typing into a text box or using a microphone. Typing or speaking while with a group of people who are near you means that all can hear what you say, and respond to it, much like a chat room. Unlike real life, where your ears allow you to localize people's voices, if you are reading text on your screen or hearing a speaker through earphones, you may not realize you have been spoken to. Therefore, Dr. Toth-Cohen teaches her students to always type or say the name of the person they are addressing to minimize miscommunication. In addition, it is good form to ensure that your microphone is not turned on during events. For example, I heard Dr. Toth-Cohen speak at a special disabilities conference held on Virtual Ability Island (http://www.virtualability.org/default.aspx) in Second Life, and an avatar in the audience who had not turned off his or her microphone transmitted distracting radio and cat sounds.

This platform brings a whole host of new ways to be polite or impolite; it is very easy to wear unprofessional clothes and make noises that would be considered rude. Users representing a real-world organization need to comply with proper rules of conduct so as not to reflect poorly on their organization. In addition, users must be tolerant of avatars of all shapes, sizes, genders, species, and belief systems. Finally, users have the option of creating a profile providing information about themselves; reading their profiles can facilitate your interactions with them.

Caveats on Internet Communication

No chapter on Internet behavior would be complete without some warning about the potential for harm. Having an electronic presence makes it

> Occupational therapy practitioners' ability to communicate effectively using the Internet will have a profound effect on their future as individual practitioners and on the profession as a whole.

possible for others to steal your identity and do other things that can cost you time, money, and your personal reputation. Netiquette rules are suggestions, but Internet safety is a must. This section briefly summarizes the wealth of information from reliable sources that can help you stay safe while using the Internet (U.S. Attorney General, 2008).

Occupational therapy professionals are probably not in the habit of hiding who they are, but it is important to remember that the anonymity of online environments provides opportunities to be other than who one is in reality. Therefore, when dealing with people in online contexts, be wary and prevent difficulties by not assuming people are who they say they are.

Anything you share on the Internet may be vulnerable being seen by others. Before you share identifying information (both your own and others') with anyone, be sure the recipient can be trusted. People who would like to steal your identity can produce e-mails and Web sites that look legitimate and official. *Phishing* is the term for attempts by unscrupulous people to get personal information by sending you a letter posing as your bank or other legitimate source. The best rule is to never give out your social security number, credit card or bank account numbers, passwords, or ID numbers over the Internet. If you receive an urgent e-mail from a company, contact it by phone to see if the request for information is genuine.

The icon of a lock in the lower right-hand corner of a Web page denotes a site with safety controls, and reputable companies' Web sites usually can be trusted, but if you have any doubt, check first before you release personal information. The AOTA Web site is protected from leaks of information, so it is safe for you to share personal information there.

Communicating Appropriately and Effectively

Occupational therapy practitioners' ability to communicate effectively using the Internet will have a profound effect on their future as individual practitioners and on the profession as a whole. Netiquette offers guidelines for professional behavior in digital environments. The Internet is a wonderful tool for bringing people together throughout the world, and our ability to take advantage of the opportunities if offers to promote our profession and ourselves, and collaborate effectively with our clients (Verdonck & Ryan, 2008) will help determine the future of occupational therapy.

Thanks to Tina Champagne, OTD, for her input in the discussion groups section and to Dr. Susan Toth-Cohen for her contribution to the virtual contexts section.

REFERENCES

Babiss, F. (2007). Using new technologies to promote occupational therapy. *OT Practice, 12*(6), 17–18, 20–22, 25.

Chomsky, N. (2002, October 16). Peace netter [Interview of Noam Chomsky by Hamish Mackintosh]. *The Guardian.* Retrieved from http://www.guardian.co.uk/technology/2002/oct/17/internetnews.interviews

Goleman, D. (1997). *Emotional intelligence: Why it can matter more than IQ.* New York: Bantam.

Goleman, D. (2007, October 7). E-mail is easy to write (and to misread). *New York Times.* Retrieved July 7, 2011, from http://www.nytimes.com/2007/10/07/jobs/07pre.html?ref=danielgoleman

Hambridge, S. (1995). *Netiquette guidelines.* Retrieved July 8, 2011, from http://tools.ietf.org/html/rfc1855

Lancaster, L. C., & Stillman, D. (2002). *When generations collide: Who they are. Why they clash. How to solve the generational puzzle at work.* New York: Harper Business.

Morriss, A. P. (1998). The Wild West meets cyberspace. *The Freeman, 48*(7). Retrieved July 4, 2011, from http://www.thefreemanonline.org/featured/the-wild-west-meets-cyberspace

Shea, V. (1997). *Netiquette.* Retrieved July 2, 2010, from http://www.albion.com/netiquette/book/index.html

Shipley, D., & Schwalbe, W. (2007). *Send: The essential guide to email for office and home.* New York: Knopf.

Thompson, S. (2007). *Proper Internet forum and message board etiquette.* Retrieved August 8, 2010, from http://www.associatedcontent.com/article/160559/proper_internet_forum_and_message_board.html?cat=4

Tomlinson, R. (n.d.). *The first network email.* Retrieved July 4, 2011, from http://openmap.bbn.com/~tomlinso/ray/firstemailframe.html

U.S. Attorney General. (2008). *Internet safety: Adults.* Retrieved August 15, 2010, from http://www.atg.wa.gov/InternetSafety/Adults.aspx

Verdonck, M. C., & Ryan, S. (2008). Mainstream technology as an occupational therapy tool: Technophobe or technogeek? *British Journal of Occupational Therapy, 71,* 253–256.

Wikipedia. (2011a). *Netiquette.* Retrieved July 7, 2011, from http://en.wikipedia.org/wiki/Netiquette

Wikipedia. (2011b). *Web 2.0.* Retrieved July 7, 2011, from http://en.wikipedia.org/wiki/Web?_2.0

Yale University Library. (2007). *Staff training and organizational development: Email netiquette.* Retrieved August 4, 2010, from http://www.library.yale.edu/training/netiquette/

Sharing Your Writing Knowledge

Teaching Others to Write

RONDALYN V. WHITNEY, PhD, OT/L

For good teaching rests neither in accumulating a shelf full of knowledge nor in developing a repertoire of skills. In the end, good teaching lies in a willingness to attend and care for what happens in our students, ourselves, and the space between us. Good teaching is a certain kind of stance, I think. It is a stance of receptivity, of attunement, of listening.

—Laurent A. Daloz (1986)

By the time I entered college, I was a reporter for my hometown newspaper and had my own weekly editorial column. I had won a scholarship to Brown University's summer journalism program, which included an internship at the *New York Times*. I had won the English award. I had had two poems published and two summer internships under Pulitzer Prize–winning journalists. I was 16. I tested out of freshman English and was invited to honors English. Thinking it would be an easy A, I took freshman English and met, for the first time in my life, the brick wall of deflating feedback on my writing. It was a real discouragement for me, and I never took another English class again.

As computer science professor Randy Pausch (2007) said in his *Last Lecture*, "Some brick walls are made of flesh." The lesson, as he put it, is to see if you want something bad enough to dismantle the brick wall. Teaching can inspire fear and angst in budding writers, but some inspires great writing. Teaching should be an entryway, not a wall of brick.

> **The art of teaching is in large part the art of giving feedback that instructs but does not deflate and that motivates even the most hesitant writer to give it a go.**

Writing well is a discipline that is challenging, rewarding, and simplified by practice. Finding your voice as a writer can become an artistic, satisfying act, one that will open you up to a life of reflection and self-expression. Teaching others to write is a discipline, a masterful orchestration that changes routines, behavior, habits of thought, and the practice of putting pen to page. Although developing proficiency in writing takes time and practice, proficiency in teaching others to write is constructed through experience and knowledge. The art of teaching is in large part the art of giving feedback that instructs but does not deflate and that motivates even the most hesitant writer to give it a go. Not everyone who can write can teach well. Not everyone who can teach has learned to write well. They are two distinct skill sets, each with its own mastery.

Too many students tell me they are convinced they can't write. They use past teacher comments as evidence of their own woeful ineptitude. I'm confident that no teacher meant to cause this festering self-doubt. Writing, it seems, has a reputation as something you're either good at or you're not, and the path to getting better seems arbitrary, humbling, and sometimes insurmountable. Instructors can inadvertently compound a preexisting sensitivity. One student summed it up: "Writing class was a game of 'guess what's in my head.' You got a 'yes' or a 'no' on your paper, and you went home to guess again."

Good instruction and good feedback create an on-ramp to mastery. College writing courses, in particular those for health care professionals and non–English majors, are designed to instill the craft of writing as a means of communicating professional ideas. To follow best practices related to writing, instruction needs to be a lighthearted, playful romp with words and ideas if professionals are to use it as a tool to expand the profession's knowledge.

None of my ideas about meeting that goal are unique; any good instruction about writing says basically the same thing I have to say. I have certainly pulled from many sources; generations of teachers and writing coaches have discovered and recommended similar directions in the past. Nevertheless, this chapter presents my version, field-tested in my own writing and in the classes I have taught and tailored to the needs of aspiring health care professionals.

Over the years, I have grown confident in my belief that everyone has something valuable to share, can learn how to bring their ideas forward in written form, and has the capacity to write powerfully and with great skill. Many of us just need a little encouragement, a structure, or a reason to make the effort.

I knew I wanted to write even as a young undergraduate. I pursued writing courses under published authors and poetry workshops under masterful poets and benefitted from astute feedback from those who were committed to my writing being excellent. They encouraged my passion to write while correcting my technique. I have enjoyed writing a book, being an editor, writing for an assortment of magazines, writing chapters for publications of the American Occupational Therapy Association, and having poems published in literary publications. I guess my passion for teaching writing is a form of paying forward all the support I have received for writing over the years.

The first professional piece I published was in *OT Practice,* a continuing education article on nonverbal learning disorders (Whitney, 2004). I used a full ream of paper and stressed over the article until my husband said, "You're an expert on this subject; just tell them what you know." I'd been working so hard to say it "right" that I had thwarted myself. The *OT Practice* editor I worked with seemed to understand that writing scares professionals more than it scares novices because a professional career rides on what one writes. In each round of her feedback, I felt invited to do more writing for my profession rather than feeling silenced. I have since sat on several working committees with this editor, and although she seems to have no memory of that earliest interaction, I remember her with respect and admiration and think of her as one who opened a door for me and helped me walk through.

Many others share my passion for encouraging writers and writing instruction. I can't say enough about the efforts of the National Writing Project (NWP), a national program to improve the writing achievement of students across grade levels, schools, and contexts and to teach instructors evidence-based strategies to help students become accomplished writers (see http://www.nwp.org/). The NWP is the largest-scale and longest-standing teacher development program in U.S. history and provides workshops, resources, and support for anyone who wishes to teach writing. The

NWP has sites in universities across the country providing workshops and support for teachers who wish to improve writing instruction in their schools. Some NWP sites offer special writing programs for children. If you're planning to teach people to write, I suggest you avail yourself of NWP's vast body of knowledge and willing support.

The suggestions in this chapter are not for everyone. Many teachers or editors will find this advice to be old hat. If your strategies are successful but the polar opposite of mine, by all means ignore my suggestions. I encourage you to take anything that seems new or useful here and leave the rest. And if your approach is unproductive or unsatisfying, if your students still aren't writing well and you are frustrated by that, then perhaps you are ready to take a step outside your comfort zone and try something new.

Creating an On-Ramp for Emerging Writers: Providing Structured, Focused Practice

As Heinlein's (1988) character Lazarus Long said in *Time Enough for Love,* "Never try to teach a pig to sing. It wastes your time and annoys the pig." Instructors need to understand where their students are and what they are capable of learning. This understanding is necessary to a developmental approach to teaching and helps instructors avoid expectations that will ultimately waste their time and annoy both them and their students.

Writers are developing a skill, and teaching writing requires that instructors support development that builds the essential foundational skills. Like lasers, which are powerful because they focus their energy on a small target, writing assignments that allow students to focus on and master specific skills can be more powerful than those that take a broad-stroke approach. Targeting specific skills for students to focus on also helps instructors establish a clear context for grading and critique.

REFLECTION PAPERS

For the writing course I taught, I assigned reflection papers as practice. I asked students to read about and reflect on five specific topics (see Box 18.1 for topics and assigned readings) and prepare a 1- to 2-page reflection paper on each, focusing on their writing skills. These reflection papers gave me

BOX 18.1.

TOPICS FOR THE REFLECTION PAPER ASSIGNMENTS

Reflection Paper 1: Thesis Statement

Read the Web page on how to write a thesis statement at http://www.unc.edu/depts/wcweb/handouts/thesis.html, and write a 1- to 2-page paper on your thoughts, interpretation, and learning from this source (Writing Center, University of North Carolina at Chapel Hill, n.d.).

Reflection Paper 2: Sensory Vocabulary and Observation Skills

Using the form in your course reader, fill out the page on observations related to the senses [see Figure 4.1, this volume], and write a reflection paper about this process.

Reflection Paper 3: Revision

Read the Web page on revision at http://www.unc.edu/depts/wcweb/handouts/revision.html, and write a 1- to 2-page paper on your thoughts, interpretation, and learning on the topic of revision.

Reflection Paper 4: Unusual Finding in Classroom

We will have an activity in class, and afterward you are to write about the topic, demonstrating understanding of the three-drawer technique.

Reflection Paper 5: Tech Museum Visit

Attend the Body Worlds exhibit, and write about that experience as informed by your class reading from *Stiff: The Curious Lives of Human Cadavers* (Roach, 2003).

baseline information about the students' writing ability and material I could use to provide them with feedback. I explained that each paper must contain the following elements:

- Strong thesis statement at the end of the first paragraph

- Three (no more, no fewer) details in the thesis statement

- Discussion of those three details, in order, in the body of the paper

- Three points of elaboration (no more, no fewer) in the discussion of each detail

- Conclusion that asks a question or makes a comment, such as sharing insight to the writer's opinion. For example, a student once wrote the following thesis statement:

> The best part of watching the movie *An Inconvenient Truth* was my king sized box of Junior Mints, receiving a Red Eagle Feather from an older, Native American man from the Cherakawa tribe and learning to reach, three times, for transformation.

Then, the student's conclusion comment was

> I'm still not convinced Al Gore can transform committed polluters into transforming capitalistic habits and reducing their ecofootprint but I do know having the opportunity to talk with a Cherakawa tribe leader about his life's journey transformed my ideas of how I can live my life in a way that honors the spirit of the earth.

- Rich sensory vocabulary (for extra points).

I explained to students that teaching them to write well was a survival tactic for me—reading 25 well-written 20-page scholarly papers at the end of the semester was much easier than trying to slog through 25 terribly written papers. It was in my best interest to get them organized and writing well and to let them know I had a vested interest in their success. The organizational structure, a clear grading rubric (Figure 18.1), and early and intense feedback gave students a clear chance to win.

GRADING EXPECTATIONS

The reflection paper assignments provided an incentive for students to write well, and the grading rubric I used involved little penalty for those lower on the learning curve. The grading rubric reflected a developmental approach in its assumption that students would get better by incorporating the feedback I gave them on the reflection papers and applying that feedback when they wrote the lengthier, more weighted papers in the class: a critical analysis, a 20-page scholarly paper, and a written essay in the final exam. The rubric also rewarded students who were already at a high level of mastery or who put time into the papers early on in the semester; these students were excused from completing an assignment at the very end of the course, when their other coursework intensified. Because the reflection papers were designed to be opportunities to obtain feedback and improve on

1	Provide page numbers when directly quoting a source. Not providing page numbers is considered plagiarism. When a direct quote is used, provide quotation marks around the pertinent text. If paraphrasing information from a reference source, do not provide page numbers, but be sure to provide a reference.
2	When referencing in text, list all authors in the first citation (if six or fewer), use "et al." in subsequent citations (e.g., Smith et al., 2002).
3	Reference more frequently. In a paper of this type, provide references at least every paragraph.
4	List all references cited in the text of the paper on the reference page. Cite all references listed on the reference page in the body of the text.
5	Do not cite the course reader or instructor in the paper; these are secondary sources. Confirm any information provided in the reader through a primary research source.
6	In citations in the body/text of the paper, provide author(s) last name and the year of publication only (e.g., Smith, Jones, & Fry, 2004).
7	In edited books in which chapters have individual authors, cite the chapter author, not the book editor. Refer to APA for proper format.
8	For online reference sources, cite the author or organization rather than the Web address as author. Refer to APA for proper format.
9	In referencing a publication with no date, indicate "n.d." where the year of the publication would be provided, e.g., American Cancer Society. (n.d.). or in text as (American Cancer Society, n.d.).
10	For multiple references with the same author and same year of publication (e.g., Smith published two different articles about cancer in the same year), designate each separate citation with a letter (a, b, c) to distinguish them, for example, (Smith, 2004a, 2004b).
11	This reference does not follow APA format; refer to APA for correct style.
12	Awkward sentence structure due to poor mechanics: (a) wrong preposition, (b) not a parallel construction, (c) not the right word, or (d) off topic.
13	Nonacademic tone.

Note. APA = *Publication Manual of the American Psychological Association* (2010).

FIGURE 18.1. Sample grading rubric.

> **Students need to practice writing—a lot—so they can accept feedback on their work, integrate new learning, move up the ladder, and see the results of their learning.**

common errors, students who started the course strong needed fewer feedback opportunities than those who needed some remediation. I could then reward progress and effort as they generalized to the more important assignments in the class.

Students need to practice writing—a lot—so they can accept feedback on their work, integrate new learning, move up the ladder, and see the results of their learning. The beginning of class was the baseline; I wanted to show students a pathway for improvement that would benefit them at the end of the course and beyond.

I graded the reflection papers with a check plus (3 points), check (2 points), check minus (1 point), or no points and required a total of 10 points. Students who earned at least three check plus grades could opt out of the fifth reflection paper, as they had 90% on the assignment. That way, there was an incentive to write one's best each time. These grades were based on the following expectations:

- *Check plus* = well written, no errors, student exceeded expectations
- *Check* = well written, minimum errors, student met expectations
- *Check minus* = poorly written, multiple errors, minimal effort evident, late
- *No credit* = off topic, effort below expectations, late.

If the elements I specified (i.e., introduction with thesis statement and three details, body with three points of elaboration on each detail, and conclusion) were present, and if the paper was turned in on time and was on topic, students received a check. If the paper was also free of mechanical and grammatical errors, they received a check plus. I wanted to be clear that my comments were tied directly to what I had outlined as targeted criteria for strong writing. Figure 18.2 provides examples of my feedback form.

The reflection papers provided a structure for showing students how A papers could add creativity and move to A+ and B papers could true up to technique and move to an A. In the margins of their papers, I sometimes wrote notes or comments in a sort of running conversation with the student. I might write, "Something brilliant needs to go here" or "Made me laugh" or "I loved this!" or "Use sensory vocabulary here." I tried to make

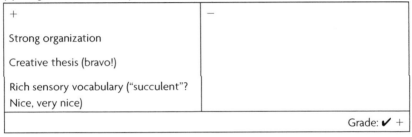

(a) Assignment meets expectations

+	—
Good organization Strong thesis Rich sensory vocabulary	More than 3 mechanical errors (review use of commas and prepositions, and add the errors to your common errors checklist) Typos (you need to proofread)
	Grade: ✔

(b) Assignment exceeds expectations

+	—
Strong organization Creative thesis (bravo!) Rich sensory vocabulary ("succulent"? Nice, very nice)	
	Grade: ✔ +

Figure 18.2. Sample feedback forms for the reflection paper assignments: (a) Assignment meets expectations; (b) Assignment exceeds expectations.

my comments lighthearted. I might pontificate on million-dollar words to encourage expansion of vocabulary; for example,

> "The coffee was hot, smelled good, and woke you all up"–really? Is that the best you've got? How about "The coffee was scorching, smoldering, a busy cauldron of a brew" or "The whiff of coffee seemed ubiquitous, the black liquid a transformative elixir restoring hordes of zombies to college freshmen"?

By now, you are likely scratching your head and wondering how I graded all this writing I asked students to produce. I made grading simple for myself by using a grading sheet that allowed me to codify my feedback. Instead of writing "You need a citation here" 25 times, I used a code and provided students with a legend. I got the idea for this shortcut from Alison George, a skilled lecturer at San José State's Occupational Therapy Department, and expanded it for my classes. I used a consistent template so my critique would be concise, organized, and targeted, as in the examples in Figure 18.2. You can develop more complicated rubrics using the free online tool Rubi-Star (see http://rubistar.4teachers.org/).

Critical Analysis Paper (50 points)		
Criterion	**Comments**	**Grade**
Organization (10 points)	The body of your paper does not follow your thesis statement.	9/10
Mechanics (10 points)	Common error (an error a student makes often): review	8/10
APA format (20 points)	Review citation of paraphrases vs. direct quotes	19/20
Addressed topic of critique (10 points)	Positively sublime	10/10
	Total grade	46/50 = 92%
Other Comments		
+		
Nice sensory vocabulary; loved the "blinkers on a horse" analogy		
Excellent conclusion; good summation without directly repeating your thesis statement		
−		
Review online exercises at http://www.unc.edu/depts/wcweb/handouts/thesis.html and http://www.dianahacker.com/writersref/		

Note. APA = *Publication Manual of the American Psychological Association* (APA, 2010).

FIGURE 18.3. Sample grading sheet for longer assignments.

For longer assignments, I had a more robust rubric but still contained my grading to the grading sheet (see Figure 18.3 for an example) and wrote comments in the margin of the paper. The rubric included comments on organization, mechanics, American Psychological Association (APA, 2010) format, and skill in addressing the topic. I used the concept of "picking up points off the table"—easy points that were to be had by following the rules for the assignment, staying on topic, proofreading and correcting errors and typos, turning in the assignment on time, and making the presentation professional. These are basic requirements, and I told students that fulfilling them would earn them half credit on an assignment.

Some students were upset if they followed the basics but received a marginal grade; others didn't seem to realize that grammar and mechanics

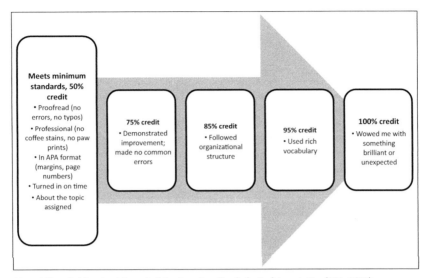

Note. APA = *Publication Manual of the American Psychological Association* (APA, 2010).

Figure 18.4. Student handout illustrating criteria for grading writing assignments.

would count. So I offered them a graphic, shown in Figure 18.4, specifying minimal expectations and illustrating how to raise their grade.

Giving Feedback: Critique Rather Than Criticism

Feedback needs to be encouraging but also to tell the truth, and walking the fine line between critique and criticism is an incomparable art. The distinction between *critique*—a detailed evaluation—and *criticism*—a list of shortcomings—is an important one, and if students can distinguish critique from criticism, they're on their way to accepting feedback and growing as writers. Teachers help them learn by modeling giving constructive feedback, having students practice giving feedback, and modeling acceptance of critique.

MODEL GIVING CONSTRUCTIVE FEEDBACK

Writing is a form of thinking, and if teachers judge students' writing harshly, we risk personally attacking their innermost thoughts. Our feedback as editors, instructors, and coaches should be about the writing, not the person and not the ideas. For example, instead of "That's boring," a constructive critique would be, "You need to develop your idea more" or "I'm feeling lost and need you to organize this section" or even "Use more sensory vocabulary here to spice this section up!" One student shared her experience of writing an essay in middle school. She had recently lost her father and had written an essay about a cat that had wandered into her life on the same day and served, somehow, as a substitute for her father's love. In large red letters, the teacher had written, "You're weird." If the piece had been off topic or wordy, a low grade might have been appropriate, but a B— and "You're weird" insulted her thoughts, feelings, and willingness to take a risk in self-expression.

Feedback needs to be gentle but instructive—an invitation to write better, not a whip of belittlement. Insensitive feedback leads to constant vigilance and defensive writing, which are bad for the spirit and a sure invitation to writer's block. *Writing defensively* means not taking risks in expressing complicated thoughts or feelings and unique connections, and it will not lead to excellence (Elbow, 2008). If each act of writing makes us fear a painful blow, we will wince and cower, and we will not be moved to write, on purpose, when no one is forcing us to do so. The risk needs to be low enough to try and high enough to be motivating. Students must experience the writing process as Fred Astaire experienced dancing: as an opportunity to be graceless on a newly set stage. Instructors set the stage, put out various props, and encourage expression in a risky leap or unexpected turn of phrase. I once had a student write an essay that began, "My cat would taste like gnocchi"—risky, but good, writing.

> Students must experience the writing process as Fred Astaire experienced dancing: as an opportunity to be graceless on a newly set stage. Instructors set the stage, put out various props, and encourage expression in a risky leap or unexpected turn of phrase.

Asking students to write a lot and finding grading schemes that make it manageable for you to give them good feedback help reconstruct their associations with red ink from enemy to friend. One important part of teaching writing is to teach students the importance of finding a good coach, editor, or peer reviewer, of trusting that person and using his or her feedback to make their writing better. Writing teachers have to instill and model this message: You have to trust people to treat you right and tell you the truth, and listening to them will help you improve your writing.

HAVE STUDENTS PRACTICE GIVING FEEDBACK

In-class practice can help students grow comfortable both giving and receiving feedback. For example, in my writing course each student brought in an idea for his or her scholarly paper and shared the idea with the class. Their classmates then shared one thing they liked about the idea and one thing they thought would improve it. Or we went around the class and each classmate contributed a comment beginning, "I want to know." Students gave me lots of positive feedback on this activity.

I also asked students to be their own critic. I assigned them the task of gathering their most common errors, keeping a running chart, and working to solve the errors. The midterm was a paper in APA format about the errors they made at the beginning of class, how they resolved them, and the resources they used to overcome the errors (e.g., Strunk & White, 2000; Truss, 2004). They had to use at least three references to scholarly publications, so a student who was not a native English speaker, for example, might discuss a study showing that students whose primary language is other than English struggle with prepositions and then describe how he or she practiced prepositions during the semester. They were required to include their common error checklist and to demonstrate that they used it when proofing their own papers.

MODEL ACCEPTANCE OF CRITIQUE

Teaching writing is a therapeutic use of self: teacher as coach and inspirer. If we are to teach our students to accept feedback, we need to model acceptance of critique and show them how to differentiate critique from criticism. I taught these important lessons using the evolving drafts of a chapter I wrote, including the planning stage, the writing phase, the revision stage, and the editing and review stage. (I'm not immune to ego bruising, so I also share the polished published work!) Students cannot imagine what a work was like before it was ready for publication. New writers need to see writing as it unfolds, while the writing is rough and unpolished, and to realize that good writers rewrite—a lot (Becker, 1986; Elbow, 2008). Sharing less-polished work by published authors is a uniquely valuable teaching tool; students thrive in the presence of those who have gone before (Zachary, 2000).

I gave each draft in turn to students to practice critiquing others' work (I do not tell them it is my work, only that it is a published author, but some guess the truth). They were very harsh! We moved through the drafts together, in small groups, and watched the piece evolve. By the end, the students had seen the dynamic movement of planning, writing, revising, editing, and proofing, as well as the final work. The process was normalizing, and the on-ramp to success began to seem less steep. In this process, I strengthened my own tolerance for the risk of exposure to reveal the habits of writing. It was a leap of faith, but the students never let me fall, and in fact we all became stronger during this exchange. They learned to be less harsh in critique and to be more open to revision. The class session often unfolded into a dialogue about the rituals of writing, like lighting a candle when you're working and blowing it out when you're done with that piece, or collecting words or favorite writers or inspiring works. I ended the class by passing out the poem "Why I Am Not a Painter" by Frank O'Hara (2008), a poem about what can happen in revision.

One other practice I used to model—acceptance of critique—was to request feedback about the class itself. Daily, as part of the requirement for class participation, I asked the students to write their name and an indication of their participation on an index card; if they had participated aloud, they could just write, "I commented," and if not, they could still "participate" by asking a clarifying question, commenting on something from the class, or asking for more information. They turned the cards in before leaving class. I learned a lot about a class this way—what I thought I covered well but didn't, what the students found helpful, and how each student gave feedback. I even used the final exam as a way to gather feedback: I required them to reflect on the course itself and to tell me what they learned. I usually structured it like this:

1. Using good organizational structure, tell me three things you've learned this semester that have improved your writing.
2. Identify two of your favorite assignments in this class. Assume I am going to get rid of them, and persuade me to keep them for future students.
3. Using rich sensory vocabulary, tell me one thing that could make this course better.

I took a risk, for sure, but I got some pretty good critique from the students that has made me a better instructor over the years.

Other Assignments to Give Students Practice Writing

Writer's block is a form of cognitive dissonance, of the moment when we experience the uncomfortable tension resulting from having two conflicting thoughts at the same time, such as "This has to sound smart" and "I can't think of anything smart to say!" Writers write by kinesthetic methods; otherwise, they are only thinkers. Writing requires the movement of a pen scratching across a page or fingers moving and translating tapping into font. This force of momentum cannot be overstated: You have to start moving body parts to get your ideas moving.

The purpose of taking a course on writing, again, is to practice writing, get feedback, and learn that you really can write about anything and that ideas are indeed everywhere, even in your own backpack or pocket. Playful activities that are rich writing experiences like those described in this section help students practice moving the pen. Some of the best student papers I have ever read came from assignments meant to budge immobility.

FLUENCY PRACTICE

Learning to write with fluency can be a challenge. Helping students practice in-class fluency, at-home fluency, and fluency in work that starts in class but is completed at home gives them the opportunity to practice in each context. Let me give you an example of each.

For in-class fluency, I hand out a 12-inch piece of string and say, "This is your lasso for an idea." I guide the students in tying the string together to make a circle, talk about observing up close and from afar, and describe the importance of "bounding" one's field of vision. For example, I can throw the circle on the ground and see gum, a blade of grass, or a cigarette butt, or I can hold it up and see clouds in the April sky. Then I send the students outside for 20 minutes. They are to drop their circle or hold it up and write down everything (*everything*) they see in the bounded circle. When they return to class, they write an in-class reflection paper on their observations following the organizational structure we're practicing. I often use this assignment when spring fever strikes.

Writing bursts are another fluency exercise I use. Everyone takes out a sheet of paper. They have 2 minutes to think of a topic—for example, autumn—and write it at the top. Then they pass it to the student on their left. That student has 1 minute to write down three details (e.g., colorful, cooler, barren) and pass it to their left. The next student writes three elaborations on the first detail (colorful—orange, radiant, fleeting), then they pass it on. The next student writes elaborations on the second detail (chilled to the bone, boundary of winter, pumpkins) and the next student on the third (empty, empty nest, toothless). The next student writes a question or makes a summarizing comment (This year, I will miss my mother's pumpkin soup). The last student receives the paper scribbled with thoughts and has 15 minutes to write a working thesis statement and a reflection on the topic. The student who completes the assignment gets the grade.

Thus, in this example, seven students write, in rapid sequence and in a very small amount of time, about seven topics that may be wildly different. The exercise shows students that they can write about anything if they follow the technique, that writing can be fun even when random, and that writing doesn't have to be serious or take forever.

Outside of class, I might assign a sensory vocabulary exercise using a format similar to the one shown in Box 18.2. Students pick an object in their environment and observe it. They describe it using each sensory pathway—how it looks, sounds, feels, moves, tastes, and smells. They then write their essay following the three-drawer technique (described in the next section) and bring their paper back to class. Later in the course, on any assignment, I ask them to include, during the planning phase, a short

---

BOX 18.2.
WORDS ORGANIZED BY SENSES

Vision	size, shape, color (e.g., round, irregular, blue)
Smell/taste	pleasant, stinky (e.g., rank, pumpkiny, spicy, putrid)
Location (proprioception)	above, below, underneath
Hearing	loud, soothing (e.g., harmonious, melodic, jarring)
Touch	texture, temperature (e.g., silky, scratchy, arctic, warm)

Tip: Before writing, make a list of relevant vocabulary you want to include or may want to include in your essay.

list of vocabulary words they will use in their essay, with a concentration on sensory words.

The assignment used to teach fluency starting in class and continuing at home is an odd but very engaging task. I introduce a novel idea by asking students to pull something out of their purse or backpack that they think no one else in the class has. I then ask each student to share their "found object." We narrow them down to the three weirdest objects, and I send each owner to the board. Three teams work to identify three details and three elaborations about the object, along with five sensory words describing it. As a class, we vote on the object that is most interesting or easiest to write about, and the students complete one of their assigned reflection papers on that object.

ORGANIZATION PRACTICE: THE THREE-DRAWER TECHNIQUE

Most people organize their clothes in the dresser as follows: underwear and socks in the first drawer, shirts in the second, and pants in the third. In 15 years of asking about this, I've met only five people who organize their clothes differently. I ask students to tell me what they keep in their top, middle, and bottom drawers, and everyone is amazed that they all answer the same. Then I point out that we all understand organization—in dressing, we move from inside to outside, then top to bottom. Writing, I explain, has a similar logic in organization: The thesis statement provides the foundation and goes in the top drawer; the body of the paper, in the middle drawer, elaborates on the elements of the thesis (which I call the *details*); and in the bottom drawer is the summary or conclusion.

In assignments using the three-drawer technique, I have students name three topics in the top drawer—their thesis statement. In the middle drawer, or body, students elaborate on those three topics with three supporting details, using sensory words when possible to enliven the text. To illustrate, the following is a brief outline of Chapter 4 of this volume using the three-drawer technique:

- *Top drawer (thesis statement):* Writers need to update the tools in their toolkit, to follow a process for using those tools to communicate effectively, and to improve their skills over time.
- *Middle drawer (supporting details with elaboration):* (1) the tools in a writer's toolkit—words, sentences, paragraphs/sections; (2) the process for using those tools to communicate effectively—five-step process,

slashers/bashers, tone; and (3) a way to improve skills over time—feedback, common errors, organized outline.

- *Bottom drawer (conclusion revisiting the thesis statement):* Strengthening your toolkit, following the writing process, and sleuthing out and eliminating errors will help you refresh, renew, and remediate your writing.

This three-drawer technique is used very successfully by students. I developed it with students I treated who had written expression disorders, and I've successfully used it with third-grade students and older.

The three-drawer technique can also be used to teach students, as I put it, "How to eat an elephant." You've heard the old joke: How do you eat an elephant? One bite at a time. Writing a long paper feels scary to students and novice writers, but breaking it down visually can really help. Table 18.1 provides an example of how to organize a 20-page paper page by page using the three-drawer technique. I write each page number on the board and lead students in filling out their outlines. If they're writing a group paper, this outline helps them divide the work more easily—one detail and elaboration per group member, for example. With this visual outline, all of a sudden the paper doesn't look so overwhelming; the students just use the same organization they've used in practice assignments all semester.

PLAYFUL ASSIGNMENTS IN THE AGE OF GOOGLE

With the Internet, cheating and plagiarism are real issues in writing classes. I get ahead of the problem by assigning papers no one can borrow from another. For example, you can't do a Google search and find a paper on the topic of "a shiny ballerina pen found in my classmate's backpack." One semester I had a student whose negative attitude really was a block to the class process, and he was gaining no friends. He was prone to rant about anything. I assigned an in-class 7-minute rant to be written using the technique we had discussed. He started laughing and wrote the best paper in the class that day. Being spontaneous and using some creativity can keep the course lively and also prevent students from finding canned papers on the Web.

> **Writing a long paper feels scary to students and novice writers, but breaking it down visually can really help.**

TABLE 18.1. Contents of a 20-Page Paper Organized Using the Three-Drawer Technique

Page	Contents
1	Introduction
2	Introduction
3	Detail 1
4	Elaboration 1 on Detail 1
5	Elaboration 2 on Detail 1
6	Elaboration 3 on Detail 1
7	Extra space to accommodate text overflow, graph, table, and/or a long quote for Detail 1
8	Detail 2
9	Elaboration 1 on Detail 2
10	Elaboration 2 on Detail 2
11	Elaboration 3 on Detail 2
12	Extra space to accommodate text overflow, graph, table, and/or a long quote for Detail 2
13	Detail 3
14	Elaboration 1 on Detail 3
15	Elaboration 2 on Detail 3
16	Elaboration 3 on Detail 3
17	Extra space to accommodate text overflow, graph, table, and/or a long quote for Detail 3
18	Conclusion
19	Conclusion
20	A brilliant insight, stated as a question or comment

One year, I had the students read an excellent example of a well-written book about an extremely odd topic. Mary Roach's (2003) book *Stiff: The Curious Lives of Human Cadavers* is a wonderful illustration of how you really can write about anything. The assignment was to read the book and create a small-group presentation related to one of the chapters. That semester the Body Worlds exhibit came to town, and our students could go for free. I required a trip to the exhibit and assigned the trip as a topic for one of the reflection papers.

Teaching Others to Write

Words have power to change ideals, shift paradigms, and influence policy. Teachers of writing invite students into the power and joy of writing and future professionals into the circle of lifelong communicators via the written word. Each time our students publish, our own contribution to the profession ripples outward. Lighthearted activities that include well-orchestrated practice and feedback help future writers ride a swell of empowerment to share their discoveries.

REFERENCES

American Psychological Association. (2010). *Publication manual of the American Psychological Association* (6th ed.). Washington, DC: Author.

Becker, H. (1986). *Writing for social scientists: How to start and finish your thesis, book, or article.* Chicago: University of Chicago Press.

Daloz, L. A. (1986). *Effective teaching and mentoring.* San Francisco: Jossey-Bass.

Elbow, P. (2008). *Writing with power: Techniques for mastering the writing process* (2nd ed.). New York: Oxford University Press.

Heinlein, R. (1988). *Time enough for love.* New York: Ace Books.

O'Hara, F. (2008). Why I am not a painter. In *Selected poems* (p. 113). New York: Knopf.

Pausch, R. (2007). *The last lecture.* Retrieved July 2, 2011, from http://www.cmu.edu/uls/journeys/randy-pausch/index.html

Roach, M. (2003). *Stiff: The curious lives of human cadavers.* New York: W. W. Norton.

Strunk, Jr., W., & White, E. B. (2000). *The elements of style* (4th ed.). Needham Heights, MA: Allyn & Bacon.

Truss, L. (2004). *Eats, shoots and leaves: The zero tolerance approach to punctuation.* New York: Gotham Books.

Whitney, R. V. (2004, December 20). Understanding nonverbal learning disorders: Nonverbal learning disability (NLD), Asperger syndrome (AS), and high-functioning autism (HFA). *OT Practice, 9*(22), CE-1–CE-8.

Writing Center, University of North Carolina at Chapel Hill. (n.d.). *Thesis statements.* Retrieved July 3, 2011, from http://www.unc.edu/depts/wcweb/handouts/thesis.html

Zachary, L. (2000). *The mentor's guide: Facilitating effective learning relationships.* San Francisco: Jossey-Bass.

RECOMMENDED READING

Ackerman, D. (1990). *A natural history of the senses.* New York: Vintage Books.

DeSalvo, L. (2000). *Writing as a way of healing: How telling our stories transforms our lives.* Boston: Beacon Press.

De Vinck, C. (1993). *Only the heart knows how to find them: Precious memories for a faithless time.* New York: Penguin.

Fox, J. (1995). *Finding what you didn't lose: Expressing your truth and creativity through poem-making.* New York: Putnam Books.

Goldberg, N. (1986). *Writing down the bones: Freeing the writer within.* Boston: Shambhala.

Rainer, T. (1978). *The new diary: How to use a journal for self-guidance and expanded creativity.* New York: St. Martin's Press.

Mentoring Others in Their Development as Writers

KAREN JACOBS, EdD, OTR/L, CPE, FAOTA, and
NANCY MacRAE, MS, OTR/L, FAOTA

*A lot of people have gone further than they thought they could because
someone else thought they could.*

—Unknown

Writing is a skill that takes practice, and with practice one can become a great writer. Once mastery is achieved, it is time to share your knowledge.

The mentoring process is a valuable tool that all occupational therapy practitioners and students have available to them. Mentoring can be formal or informal. Partnerships can be with those who have more experience than you or with peers, where collaboration and mutual support are necessary. Mentoring "is about learning and relationships" (Gilfoyle, Grady, & Nielson, 2011, p. 26). This interpersonal venture can become intense, but it can yield benefits for both the mentor and mentee.

Mentoring is simply providing assistance and support to another to help with his or her professional development. But this simple definition belies the inherent complexity in such a relationship. Time, context, and need are just a few of the variables that have to be considered. As this chapter addresses writing mentorships, the focus will be on factors involved in such partnerships.

Nine Truths of Writing

For a quarter of a century, we have been collaborating, brainstorming, and writing with each other about both occupational therapy and personal life topics. In fact, we have been reciprocal or peer mentors for each other. As we started the collaborative process to write this chapter, we realized we had shared several of the same experiences with writing over the years. We distilled from those common experiences the following nine truths:

1. *Writing takes courage.* To articulate something in writing that someone will read can be intimidating. We may be concerned that others will detect our ignorance or find a flaw in our reasoning or analysis of the data. We must have courage to overcome these self-doubts.
2. *Writing takes time.* An idea takes time to fully develop. Starting to write can be difficult; in fact, sometimes we need to start writing, take a break, and come back to it. Besides creating appropriate content, adhering to author guidelines and sequencing our thoughts logically take time, which leads to Truth 3.
3. *Writing is iterative.* Writing is circular in nature. We start with an idea, describe the idea with as many examples as possible, and end by synopsizing the idea, bringing it full circle. Getting the idea down "on paper" is what is important, whether in a digital document or an audio file. Once our thoughts are articulated, we can always come back and expand on them. We've learned not to edit too soon or too much; overediting while we're writing prevents the flow of creativity. Instead, we plan for multiple drafts. Professional writing can get us into an optimal flow experience and can be, and often is, a creative experience. But good writing always needs to flow first and then be edited.
4. *Writing can be an individual or team sport.* Writing need not be a singular affair; it can be done collaboratively. In fact, a writing project may benefit from or even depend on collaboration (see Chapter 6 in this volume). Many course assignments, even writing assignments, require group work. With the growing importance of interprofessional collaboration, being able to write with another, especially from another discipline, is a critical skill.

5. *Writing = learning.* We need to learn to write, and writing, conversely, helps us learn, heal, and grow. The process of writing clarifies our thinking and enhances our emotional and spiritual well-being.

> *Writing = learning.* **We need to learn to write, and writing, conversely, helps us learn, heal, and grow.**

6. *Writing can be a transformative experience.* Writing can stimulate our ideas, expand our knowledge of a subject, provide us with a new perspective, result in the satisfaction of seeing our name in print, and lead us to new insights about ourselves.

7. *Technology can enable writing.* Tools such as software for redlining text, visual mapping, and an online thesaurus or hardware such as computerized pens and a tape recorder all can be mechanisms for just getting down your ideas. Using software such as EndNote helps us keep track of references.

8. *Nurturing eases the process of writing.* Nurturing from others fosters our further development; it supports us in becoming clearer writers. It can occur in multiple ways, as noted later in this chapter. When nurturing supports the writing experience, its effects can be powerful.

9. *Effective writers know their audience.* Before completing a written document, we take steps to ensure that what we have written is understandable and relevant to our target audience. Knowing your audience allows you to use certain words and descriptions that will resonate with them and help them to understand quickly and clearly what you mean. Examples to highlight your intent can be relevant to their experiences.

Mentors empower writers to embrace these truths by providing validation, encouragement, and support. They provide constructive editing, endorse writers' efforts, and present them with the freedom to write, rewrite, and be more creative in the process. Mentoring writers, however, needs to be done with delicacy. Ideal mentors deliver constructive, honest feedback with tact, and perhaps humor, and offer alternatives to select from when making recommendations for revisions. Discerning when tact is necessary comes not only from experience but also from knowing the mentee as a person.

Mentoring a writer facilitates his or her ability to write through teaching and nurturing. We define *mentoring* as a reciprocal and mutually beneficial relationship between two people that facilitates the growth of one or the other or both. In practice, we adapt this relationship to the context of our needs; for example, Karen may be the mentor and Nancy the mentee in one situation and vice versa in another. Both parties in the relationship must use the reflective process to maximize their professional development. Such a process involves reviewing what has happened and thinking about how it might be improved, changed, or discarded.

Models for Mentoring Others as Writers

Maynard and Furlong (1995) described two models of mentorship: apprenticeship and competency. Beginning writers benefit most from an *apprenticeship model,* which focuses on the development of their basic writing skills, whereas the *competency model* occurs between professionals of more equal status who consult with one another about improving their skills and expertise in writing (Urish, 2004). We propose a third model: *collaborative editorship.*

Collaborative editorship consists of two or more people who work together to produce a compilation of writing. Each editor is usually assigned specific responsibilities, which are then reviewed by the other editors. Being an editor may or may not involve writing for the end product. For example, such an editor is a conductor for a symphony orchestra.

APPRENTICESHIP MODEL

An occupational therapy student in a teaching assistant position worked with Nancy on developing her leadership skills through mentor-guided specific sequential activities. One activity was to write an article on students' development of leadership skills and submit it for publication. As the student developed her writing skills, Nancy mentored her and edited multiple drafts of her article, which was eventually published in *OT Practice.* The student described the value of the mentoring experience as follows:

> As a new practitioner and recent graduate, I often found myself asking, "What difference can I make with the little experience that I have?" An experienced mentor, such as Nancy, opened my eyes to the many possibilities in the realm of occupational therapy and helped me understand that there are bountiful possibilities for growth and change. This includes presenting my personal leadership trajectory to peers, publishing in *OT Practice,* facilitating a small leadership

group consisting of my peers, and striving to be a leader in my field. Through such a nurturing mentorship, I have become a lifelong learner and can carry on the cyclical process of one day becoming a mentor for others. (K.C., MS, OTR/L)

COMPETENCY MODEL

We have been mentors for each other for 25 years, and each of us has also had multiple opportunities to edit the work of our peers. Both of these experiences are examples of the competency model. In many cases, although our colleagues' work was original and well referenced, we helped them refine and clarify it by ferreting out inconsistencies, unclear ideas, and need for examples and by providing guidance in fashioning more succinct and powerful endings that synthesized their key ideas. In addition to helping to refine their writing, mentoring instills in writers a sense of optimism that they can successfully complete their work.

Karen's experience as founding editor-in-chief of the journal *Work: A Journal of Prevention, Assessment and Rehabilitation* has allowed her to mentor numerous authors, many of whom had never published before. Her philosophy of not using the term *rejected* as a review status but instead encouraging rewrites has helped many potential authors become published authors.

COLLABORATIVE EDITORSHIP

In 1992, Nancy experienced her first collaborative editorship with three colleagues when they produced a special issue of the *American Journal of Occupational Therapy* on feminism (Froehlich, Hamlin, Loukas, & MacRae, 1992). Many of the truths we described in the introduction to this chapter became evident during this intense process. For example, courage was required of the four editors to write on the topic of feminism in 1992. At that time, the concept of feminism was not clearly understood, and it was not until the final submissions had been reviewed that the editors' title was allowed to stand. Using an inclusive way to demonstrate feminism helped in making this issue more acceptable and publishable.

It took time not only to write the individual articles but also to collect and edit the submitted manuscripts. The review process was iterative in nature. Certainly the entire experience was transformative, primarily because of the support and encouragement we gave one another.

A more recent example is our collaborative editorship of the textbook *Occupational Therapy Essentials for Clinical Competence* (Sladyk, Jacobs, & MacRae, 2010). The two of us and the third editor lived in different states, so we depended on technology to work together, along with the 40 contributing authors, to complete the manuscript. Even with technology, finalizing the book required a face-to-face work session by the three coeditors. As the process continued, we learned from one another about the specific assignments each had assumed. One of us proved to be very good at organizing the material, and we found a rhythm that allowed each of us to contribute to the text's introduction.

Mentoring Activities

The many activities that can be used in mentoring others in their writing can be categorized as teaching methodologies and nurturing activities. This section describes some of the activities we have found most useful. More experienced writers or ones of equal status have much to teach to and learn from each other. The reciprocal nature of this process fits well within a professional lifelong learning. There are times during this process when nurturing is also needed.

TEACHING

Occupational therapy professionals and aspiring practitioners teach: We teach our clients, family members, and other professionals. Teaching is an inherent part not only of occupational therapy but also of mentoring writers. To help mentees, mentors can use teaching strategies. Four strategies that we have found helpful are

- Using grading rubrics
- Journaling about concrete experiences
- Using metaphors to enhance descriptiveness
- Writing to promote healing.

Each strategy incorporates adult learning principles such as immediate application of what has been learned, the provision of some structure, meaningful feedback, and opportunities for choice to facilitate the engagement of mentees in writing (Knowles, 1990; Speck, 1996).

Using Grading Rubrics

One of the tools teachers use to facilitate and structure writing practice for students are rubrics. *Rubrics* provide structure and guideposts to a writing assignment; they list clear expectations for the assignment and criteria for assessing the results, including the relative importance of each aspect of the writing being assessed. Feedback may be recorded on a printout of the rubric to aid the writer in incorporating suggestions into the next draft.

Another example of the use of rubrics occurs with required peer editing of a clinical form of writing such as documentation. Initial ungraded efforts are provided with meaningful feedback that needs to be incorporated in the next draft. With associated peer editing, students are required to help one another by providing constructive feedback. In addition it provides peer editors with the knowledge that others have different strengths and similar problems that can be both learning and comforting lessons.

Journaling

One of the most effective formats mentors can use to encourage mentees to practice writing and reflection is *journaling*. Experience, activity, and re-flective thought are valuable sources of inspiration (Kolb, 1984), and journaling helps mentees reflect in writing on their experiences. Journals have been found to be catalysts for clinical learning (Tanner, 2006), for the transfer of knowledge, and for the development of reflective practitioners (Lasater, 2007; Nielson, Stragnell, & Jester, 2007). The good news is that technology can make journaling more easily accessible to all of us.

A useful time for reflection is after an experience, which Schon (1987) termed *reflection-on-action* (see also Buchbinder et al., 2005). Reflection can help in both the formation and summation of an experience, thus aiding in the development and solidification of learning. Writing is a primary means for this to occur. It encourages a review of what has happened, an assignation of what was most important and relevant to learning, and can guide the writer to the next appropriate steps.

Box 19.1 provides an example of guidelines mentees can use in recording journal entries. The two quotations that follow are journal entries by students in an entry-level occupational therapy class.

> **Reflection can help in both the formation and summation of an experience.**

BOX 19.1.
JOURNAL WRITING GUIDELINES

Journals are a tool for describing your experiences. In each journal entry, you need to do each of the following:

- Describe your experience. Specify the who, what, where, and when.
- Explain the meaning of the experience—the how and why.
- Think broadly about what you have encountered. How will what you experienced influence you in the future?

The length of a journal entry is not as important as the quality of thinking and reflecting you do while writing it. Thinking and reflecting are the keys to genuine learning experiences. We will meet regularly to review your entries.

Note. Adapted from Drinka and Clark (2000).

The entries describe their experiences in an interprofessional class tasked with devising and then implementing a fall reduction program for independently living elders.

Reflecting back on this session will influence my future practice because it made me realize the significance of developing group dynamics in the health care setting to provide better care for our clients. A team with good communication and respect for one another can provide more comprehensive care and thus more satisfied clients. I was surprised at the quick progression of group dynamics as compared to another group in which I am involved, where it is taking longer for the group to come together to accomplish a goal. Every group and setting I will be working in will have different dynamics, and some may be harder to develop than others. (E.O.B.)

The experience of what I learned at the assisted living facility will influence my future practice because I have learned what the role of the physician assistant is, how an occupational therapist can promote functional performance and engagement in meaningful activities for clients living in an assisted living facility, and the value of interdisciplinary teams. I have learned how physician assistants work with clients because I observed their assessments and listened to the types of questions they ask their clients. After observing and talking with clients, I learned what types of activities the facility offered. My understanding of the dynamics at the assisted living facility was promoted when I was immersed in the situations. Moreover, I believe interprofessional teams are very important for clients because it is important to know the client as a whole person to provide the best possible care. (L.W.)

Using Metaphors

A method to enhance understanding and communication, particularly in writing, is the use of metaphors, literary devices that are primary tools of thought and language. A *metaphor* is the use of one conceptual category, experience, or image to describe or define another conceptual category (Yero, n.d.).

Occupational therapy uses metaphors to describe client experiences in documentation, write for publication, and advocate for a client to a third-party payer. For example, "hungry for success" (a biological experience) or "shooting for promotion" (a hunting image) more vividly describe a person's goals for the future than simply "ambitious." Figurative uses of "fighting a battle," "extinguishing a fire," or "swimming in rough seas" conjure images of struggle and victory.

Schon (1979) observed that metaphors are a vehicle for enabling people to comprehend things that have gone wrong in their lives. Metaphors sum up what needs fixing and imply possible solutions, and as such, are important to understand in the renditions, verbal or written, of both our own lives and those of clients. Metaphors used by clients serve to provide meaning to their life stories being recounted. They easily allow the client and practitioner to understand complex ideas (Mallinson, Kielhofner, & Mattingly, 1996).

Mentors can use these devices to simplify what they know their mentees are experiencing. Metaphors such as "exploring the unknown" or "watching flowers grow" are examples they can share. A metaphor that fits the experience of the mentor is "being a tour guide."

Writing as Healing

We both believe in the healing power of writing. Writing narratives about stressful or painful experiences can be a strategy for clarifying and gaining new perspectives on the experience and can promote healing. A personal example follows from Nancy's life:

> I had a clarification of a concrete experience after a break of my femur. Karen encouraged me to make meaning of the experience by writing about my journey as a consumer of rehabilitation. For me, writing became a cathartic experience that helped me gain perspective on the accident and promoted cognitive

and emotional healing. Writing also had the outcome of informing my teaching. The following excerpt is from my published article in *Work:* "This surprise experience has educated me about the emotional, physical and spiritual recovery of a person. Being able to realize the positive attributes of the situation has helped me to regain a sense of equilibrium and an immense appreciation of all that my life gives to me. I have a profession about which I am passionate, friends and students who care about me, and a body which has shown its resilience and an ability to snap back to functionality. My recovery is not yet complete, but I look forward to a future filled with more self-knowledge, a better appreciation of the present, and an abiding faith in the connection of others." (MacRae, 2010, p. 397)

Nancy's was the first article in a regular column in *Work* entitled "Narrative Reflections on Occupational Transitions." The impetus in starting this column was to provide a forum for individuals to tell their own stories of successful transitions into, between, or out of occupations.

Louise DeSalvo (1999) spoke of this kind of writing in her book *Writing as a Way of Healing*. She noted that the writing process allows us to "discover strength, power, wisdom, depth, energy, creativity, soulfulness, wholeness" (p. 9) and described the qualities of a healing narrative as "render[ing] our experience concretely, authentically, explicitly, and with a richness of detail. It tells precisely what happened. It is accurate. It is rooted in time and in place" (p. 57). She continued, "A healing narrative links feelings to events" and "uses negative words to describe emotions and feelings in moderation; but it uses positive words, too" (p. 59).

NURTURING

To *nurture* means to educate, to cultivate, and to enable to grow, and in this chapter the word refers to a stance that contributes to the personal and professional sustenance of another person and the development of his or her writing skills. Nurturing is a bidirectional and dynamic bridge between the parties involved in the mentoring of writing. Without nurturing, mentoring cannot be as meaningful. Nurturing activities are when mentors provide guidance, the "just-right" kind of help, with reassurance that they believe their mentees can accomplish what the next set of goals are. They are sensitive to the needs, emotional or spiritual, of their mentees, and they act accordingly.

The value of nurturing is perceived by the recipient. Karen asked several of her doctoral students to describe the nurturing of mentoring, and their narratives shed light on the experience of being nurtured:

> **The value of nurturing is perceived by the recipient.**

> Without that nurturing arm around my shoulder that provided comfort and encouragement, the writing process would not be nearly as complete or emotionally satisfying for me. A writer can adequately convey her perspective after benefitting from teaching and mentoring, but only through the personal connection of a nurturing relationship will she become empowered to infuse her writing with a passion that engages the readers. (A.M.D., MS, OTR/L)

> Nurturing the iterative process of writing for this doctoral project is similar to the guidance we might give to our children or to our occupational therapy clients to find the "just-right" challenge at that time. As a child or client is learning something new, we might offer assistance for one part of the project now and another part later. As we completed sections and different drafts of our doctoral projects, we have been provided with similar guidance: a little then to improve one aspect, more now to develop another aspect. This was always done with what seemed an overall view of what was needed and appropriate at each stage of the writing process. (N.D., MS, OTR/L)

> Part of my best learning has come from not knowing what someone thinks about my writing, but letting my writing evolve. An important part of the nurturing process for me was the silent confidence that I would ultimately come to the right place, even if it took time to get there. I am extremely grateful for this, and I know that this has given me the confidence to succeed. (R.N., MS, OTR/L)

As each of these students noted, nurturing was a primary element of mentoring and a mechanism for successful writing outcomes. Safety, empowerment, comfort, the just-right time for feedback, and the just-right amount of feedback are elements they identified as important in a nurturing mentor relationship.

Guiding Others in Their Writing

Writing is a critical skill that occupational therapy practitioners and students who wish to reach their full potential must continually improve. Through the commitment of each of us to mentor others to write, the profession adds articulate members to its workforce. Occupational therapy practitioners and students with all levels of experience can gain confidence in their ability to express themselves through mentor-guided writing experiences such as journaling.

Writing is a process skill that needs to be used continually to grow and improve. Mentoring helps with this process. Using clear writing to address society's occupational needs will strengthen the reach of the profession and enable more people to experience improved quality of life.

The authors dedicate this chapter to the mentors and students who have helped us learn.

REFERENCES

Buchbinder, B., Alt, P. M., Eskow, K., Forbes, W., Hester, E., & Strick, M. (2005). Creating learning prisms with an interdisciplinary case study workshop. *Innovative Higher Education, 29,* 257–274.

DeSalvo, L. (1999). *Writing as a way of healing.* Boston: Beacon Press.

Drinka, T. J. K., & Clark, P. G. (2000). Team members as learners and teachers. In *Health care teamwork: Interdisciplinary practice and teaching* (pp. 163–176). Westport, CT: Auburn House.

Froehlich, J., Hamlin, R., Loukas, K., & MacRae, N. (Eds.). (1992). Special issue on feminism as an inclusive perspective. *American Journal of Occupational Therapy, 46*(11).

Gilfoyle, E., Grady, A., & Nielson, C. (2011). *Mentoring leaders: The power of storytelling for building leadership in health care and education.* Bethesda, MD: AOTA Press.

Knowles, M. S. (1990). *The adult learner: A neglected species* (4th ed.). Houston, TX: Gulf Publishing.

Kolb, D. A. (1984). *Experiential learning: Experience as the source of learning and development.* Englewood Cliffs, NJ: Prentice Hall.

Lasater, K. (2007). Clinical judgment development: Using simulation to create an assessment rubric. *Journal of Nursing Education, 46,* 496–503.

MacRae, N. (2010). Narrative reflections on occupational transitions. *Work, 35,* 395–397.

Mallinson, T., Kielhofner, G., & Mattingly, C. (1996). Metaphor and meaning in a clinical interview. *American Journal of Occupational Therapy, 50*(5), 338–346.

Maynard, T., & Furlong, J. (1995). Learning to teach and models of mentoring. In T. Kerry & A. S. Mayes (Eds.), *Issues in mentoring* (pp. 10–24). New York: Routledge.

Nielson, A., Stragnell, S., & Jester, P. (2007). Guide for reflection using the clinical judgment model. *Journal of Nursing Education, 46,* 513–516.

Schon, D. A. (1979). Generative metaphor: A perspective on problem-solving in social policy. In A. Ortony (Ed.), *Metaphor and thought* (pp. 459–471). Cambridge, England: Cambridge University Press.

Schon, D. A. (1987). *Educating the reflective practitioner.* San Francisco: Jossey-Bass.

Sladyk, K., Jacobs, K., & MacRae, N. (Eds.). (2010). *Occupational therapy essentials for clinical competence.* Thorofare, NJ: Slack.

Speck, M. (1996). Best practice in professional development for sustained educational change. *ERS Spectrum, 14*(2), 33–41.

Tanner, C. A. (2006). Thinking like a nurse: A research-based model of clinical judgment in nursing. *Journal of Nursing Education, 45,* 204–211.

Urish, C. (2004). Ongoing competence through mentoring. *OT Practice, 9*(3), 10.

Yero, J. L. (n.d.). *Common metaphors in "teacher talk."* Retrieved October 11, 2011, from http://www.teachersmind.com/Metaphor.html

SUGGESTED READING

Adams, K. (1998). *The way of the journal: A journal therapy workbook for healing.* Brooklandville, MD: Sidran Press.

Baldwin, C. (1992). *One to one: Self-understanding through journal writing.* New York: M. Evans & Co.

Batchelor, A. (n.d.). *How to keep a spiritual journal.* Retrieved October 11, 2011, from http://www.howtodothings.com/religion-spirituality/how-to-keep-a-spiritual-journal

Bateson, M. (1990). *Composing a life.* New York: Plume.

Cohn, M., Mehl, M., & Pennebaker, J. (2004). Linguistic markers of psychological change surrounding September 11, 2001. *Psychological Science, 15,* 687–693.

Cross, K. P. (1984). *Adults as learners.* San Francisco: Jossey-Bass.

Fox, J. (1997). *Poetic medicine: The healing art of poem-making.* New York: Jeremy P. Tarcher/Putnam.

Goldberg, N., & Guest, J. (1986). *Writing down the bones: Freeing the writer within.* Boston: Shambhala Press.

Jacobs, B. (2005). *Writing for emotional balance.* Oakland, CA: New Harbinger.

Pennebaker, J. W. (1997). *Opening up: The healing power of expressing emotion.* New York: Guilford Press.

Pennebaker, J. W. (2004). *Writing to heal: A guided journal for recovering from trauma and emotional upheaval.* Oakland, CA: New Harbinger.

Rainer, T. (1979). *The new diary: How to use a journal for self-guidance and expanded creativity.* New York: Jeremy P. Tarcher.

Turley, C. (2009). Fostering reflective practice. *Radiation Therapist, 18*(1), 66–68.

Index

Boxes, figures, and tables are indicated by b, f, and t, respectively, following page numbers.

About the Editors and Authors

Editors

Rondalyn V. Whitney, PhD, OT/L, is a prolific writer, occupational therapist, and researcher. She views writing as the artistic expression for activists. Whitney is passionate about helping others view writing as a powerful tool with which to create meaningful change; express powerful or salient ideas; and incite, inspire, inflame, or quiet the spirit across both generational and social boundaries. Her research areas of interest include telehealth, family quality of life, emotional disclosure, maternal stress, and attachment. She has held professional leadership roles for more than 20 years and is considered a visionary, innovator, and content expert in social participation, autism, maternal health, and the therapeutic use of narrative.

Christina A. Davis has been in scholarly, technical, and medical publishing since 1988, beginning in biological and chemical sciences before settling into psychology and health care. She is currently director of AOTA Press, which publishes the *American Journal of Occupational Therapy*, textbooks, assessments, Practice Guidelines, and exam preparation materials. Before arriving at AOTA in 2002, she managed the production and development of companion products to the 5th Edition of the *Publication Manual of the American Psychological Association*. Her life and publishing interests include animal rescue, elder care, historic preservation and home building, day trading, and classic British and American cars.

Authors

Marian Arbesman, PhD, OTR/L, is president of ArbesIdeas, Inc., Williamsville, NY; adjunct assistant professor in the Department of Rehabilitation Science at the State University of New York at Buffalo; and consultant with AOTA's Evidence-Based Practice Project.

Fran Babiss, PhD, OTR/L, is coordinator, Evidence-Based Practice, South Oaks Hospital, Amityville, NY, and clinical assistant professor, Stony Brook University, Stony Brook, NY. She has worked in behavioral health and administration for most of her career but is also interested in the use of computer technologies. She was the first occupational therapist to create a podcast covering mental health topics and is exploring the use of virtual worlds for education about and promotion of the profession.

Brent Braveman, PhD, OTR/L, FAOTA, is director, Department of Rehabilitation Services, University of Texas MD Anderson Cancer Center, Houston. He has practiced as an occupational therapy clinician, educator, researcher, and manager since entering the profession in 1984. Braveman is author of 34 refereed journal articles and book chapters, has presented at national and international conferences, and is author of two occupational therapy textbooks. He has a long history of volunteer service in state and national association activities, including serving as Speaker of the Representative Assembly for AOTA and on the AOTA Board of Directors.

Elizabeth Cara, PhD, OTR/L, MFT, is professor in occupational therapy, San Jose State University, San Jose, CA. She is the lead editor and coauthor of the three editions of the popular text *Psychosocial Occupational Therapy: An Evolving Practice* (Delmar Cengage, 2012). She has 23 years of experience in education and worked for 15 years as a practitioner in mental health settings. She has published and presented nationally and internationally. Cara began research on Dian Fossey in 2003, and she is currently finishing a book proposal related to Fossey. She has also revived her original psychobiographical work on artist Georgia O'Keeffe. She first joined her psychobiographers writing group in 1993.

Donna Costa, DHS, OTR/L, FAOTA, is professor (clinical), University of Utah, Salt Lake City. She earned her doctorate from the University of Indianapolis. Her research interests are in mindfulness-based interventions. She is a Fellow of AOTA and the author of two books on fieldwork education and numerous articles in *OT Practice*. She chairs the Education Special Interest Section of AOTA, is continuing education chair for the Utah Occupational Therapy Association, and serves on the editorial boards of the *Amer-*

ican Journal of Occupational Therapy and *Occupational Therapy in Health Care*. Costa is a member of Rotary International and serves on the board of directors of the RESOURCE Foundation, Carmel, IN.

Catherine Foster, BA, is research coordinator, Kennedy Krieger Institute, Center for Autism and Related Disorders, Baltimore. She earned her bachelor's degree in psychology from Goucher College and is currently earning her master of science in clinical psychology at Loyola University. Foster is interested in research on the impact of comorbid diagnoses on children with autism spectrum disorders. She has disseminated her research through various conference presentations and professional journals.

Lisa Foulke, BA, is managing editor, Allied Health CE, Gannett Education, Falls Church, VA. She has been an editor for more than 20 years.

Sharon A. Gutman, PhD, OTR, FAOTA, is associate professor, Programs in Occupational Therapy, Columbia University, NY, and is editor-in-chief of the *American Journal of Occupational Therapy*. She has authored numerous articles and books, including *Screening Adult Neurologic Populations: A Step-by-Step Instruction Manual* (AOTA Press, 2009), *Quick Reference Neuroscience for Rehabilitation Professionals: The Essential Neurologic Principles Underlying Rehabilitation Practice* (Slack, 2007), and *Living With Illness or Disability: 10 Lessons of Acceptance, Understanding, and Perseverance* (AOTA Press, 2005).

Robert G. Hess, Jr., RN, PhD, FAAN, is executive vice president, Global Programming, Gannett Healthcare Group, Falls Church, VA, which publishes nurse.com, *Today in OT,* and *Today in PT* and their Web sites, as well as continuingeducation.com. His content team develops thousands of educational activities for occupational therapy, nursing, pharmacy, medicine, and other allied health professions, awarding millions of contact hours annually. Hess is founder of the Forum for Shared Governance (www.sharedgovernance.org) and author of instruments for measuring governance in organizations nationally and internationally.

Karen Jacobs, EdD, OTR/L, CPE, FAOTA, is clinical professor and program director of the online postprofessional doctorate in occupational therapy program, Boston University. She is past president of AOTA, received AOTA's 2011 Eleanor Clarke Slagle Lectureship, and was a 2005 recipient of a Fulbright scholarship. Jacobs's research examines the interface between the environment and human capabilities, in particular the increased risk of functional limitations among university and middle school–age students, especially in notebook computing and backpack use.

Luther G. Kalb, MHS, is currently a doctoral candidate in the Department of Mental Health at the Johns Hopkins Bloomberg School of Public Health (JHBSPH) and serves as research manager in the Center for Autism and Related Disorders, as well as the Department of Medical Informatics, at the Kennedy Krieger Institute in Baltimore. He received a BA in applied psychology from the University of Baltimore and an MHS from JHBSPH. His research has appeared in prestigious scientific journals such as *Pediatrics, Journal of Abnormal Child Psychology,* and the *Journal of American Medical Informatics.*

Nancy MacRae, MS, OTR/L, FAOTA, is associate professor, Occupational Therapy Department, University of New England, Biddeford, ME, where she has taught for 23 years. She is past director of that department and past president of the Maine Occupational Therapy Association. MacRae has written on sexuality and aging and on interprofessional education and practice, and she coedited a basic occupational therapy text.

Alison B. Miller, PhD, is founder and owner of The Dissertation Coach, a coaching and consulting business dedicated to helping graduate students earn master's and doctoral degrees. She has a PhD in clinical psychology from the University of Illinois at Chicago. She is the author of *Finish Your Dissertation Once and for All! How to Overcome Psychological Barriers, Get Results, and Move on With Your Life* (American Psychological Association, 2009) and has authored journal articles in psychology and disability studies. For her own dissertation study, Miller examined how the experience of homelessness influenced dignity and worth among homeless men and women living in shelters. She frequently leads dissertation workshops at universities around the United States. She is also owner of Tiara, a company that offers coaching, leadership development, and workshops for women.

Suzanne M. Peloquin, PhD, OTR, FAOTA, is professor, School of Health Professions, University of Texas Medical Branch, Galveston. She is also the occupational therapist at a residential facility for women in recovery. She previously worked in mental health settings in Texas and West Virginia as a staff therapist and administrator. Peloquin received the AOTA 2005 Eleanor Clarke Slagle Lectureship. She has written extensively on the history and service of occupational therapy, the ethos and art of occupational therapy practice, and the unique manifestations of empathy and spirituality in the profession. Considered provocative by some and evocative by others, her work prompts a reflective response.

Winifred Schultz-Krohn, PhD, OTR/L, BCP, SWC, FAOTA, is professor of occupational therapy, San Jose State University, San Jose, CA. She has more than 30 years of experience working with children and families. She is a Fellow of AOTA, is board certified in pediatrics, and is swallow certified by the California Board of Occupational Therapy. Her scholarly interests include pediatric occupational therapy, the needs of children and families in homeless shelters, feeding problems, and neurological rehabilitation. Schultz-Krohn continues to practice in pediatric occupational therapy on a part-time basis and provides pro bono services at a family homeless shelter, where her donation of professional services was recognized with a regional Jefferson Award. She is coeditor of the 6th and 7th Editions of *Pedretti's Occupational Therapy: Practice Skills for Physical Dysfunction* (Mosby, 2013), has authored more than 20 articles and chapters, and serves on two editorial boards.

Jerilyn (Gigi) Smith, MS, OTR/L, SWC, is assistant professor, Occupational Therapy Department, San Jose State University, San Jose, CA. In addition to teaching and being the undergraduate advisor for the occupational therapy program, she continues her clinical practice in early intervention, working with children ages 0–3 years who have developmental disabilities and medical complications. Smith has written chapters on documentation, dysphagia, and mental health of older adults for internationally recognized occupational therapy textbooks. She is completing her PhD at Trident University.

Leonard G. Trujillo, PhD, OTR/L, is associate professor and chair, Department of Occupational Therapy, East Carolina University, Greenville, NC.

Before that he was associate professor and associate dean, School of Occupational Therapy, Texas Woman's University, Dallas Campus. He has been an occupational therapist for more than 35 years, with the majority of his clinical experience in the U.S. Air Force. In 2010 he became a Fellow of AOTA. He has received numerous internal and external grant awards, most recently associated with Operation Re-entry North Carolina.